T0202874

SpringerBriefs in Statistics

More information about this series at http://www.springer.com/series/8921

Takashi Sozu · Tomoyuki Sugimoto
Toshimitsu Hamasaki · Scott R. Evans

Sample Size Determination in Clinical Trials with Multiple Endpoints

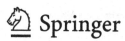 Springer

Takashi Sozu
Faculty of Engineering
Tokyo University of Science
Tokyo
Japan

Tomoyuki Sugimoto
Hirosaki University Graduate School
   of Science and Technology
Hirosaki
Japan

Toshimitsu Hamasaki
National Cerebral and Cardiovascular Center
Osaka
Japan

Scott R. Evans
Harvard T.H. Chan School of Public Health
Harvard University
Boston, MA
USA

ISSN 2191-544X   ISSN 2191-5458   (electronic)
SpringerBriefs in Statistics
ISBN 978-3-319-22004-8   ISBN 978-3-319-22005-5   (eBook)
DOI 10.1007/978-3-319-22005-5

Library of Congress Control Number: 2015946106

Springer Cham Heidelberg New York Dordrecht London

Printed on acid-free paper

Springer International Publishing AG Switzerland is part of Springer Science+Business Media
(www.springer.com)

Contents

Chapter 1
Introduction

Abstract The effects of interventions are multi-dimensional. In clinical trials, use of more than one primary endpoint offers an attractive design feature to capture a more complete characterization of the intervention effects and provide more informative intervention comparisons. For these reasons, use of more than one primary endpoint has become a common design feature in clinical trials for disease areas such as oncology, infectious disease, and cardiovascular disease. In medical product development, multiple endpoints are utilized as "co-primary" or "multiple primary" to evaluate the effects of the new interventions for the treatment of Alzheimer disease, irritable bowel syndrome, acute heart failure, and diabetes mellitus. "Co-primary" in this setting means that the trial is designed to evaluate if the intervention is superior to the control on *all* of the endpoints. In contrast, a trial with "multiple primary" endpoints is designed to evaluate if the intervention is superior to the control on *at least one* of the endpoints. In this chapter, we describe the statistical issues in clinical trials with multiple co-primary or primary endpoints. We then briefly review recent methodological developments for power and sample size calculations in these clinical trials.

Keywords Intersection-union problem · Multiple co-primary endpoints · Multiple primary endpoints · Type I error adjustment · Type II error adjustment · Union-intersection problem

The determination of sample size and the evaluation of power are fundamental and critical elements in the design of a clinical trial. If a sample size is too small then important effects may not be detected, while a sample size that is too large is wasteful of resources and unethically puts more participants at risk than necessary.

Most commonly, a single endpoint is selected and then used as the basis for the trial design including sample size determination, interim data monitoring, and final analyses. However, many recent clinical trials have utilized more than one primary endpoint. The rationale for this is that use of a single endpoint may not provide a comprehensive picture of the intervention's multidimensional effects.

For example, a major ongoing HIV treatment trial within the AIDS Clinical Trials Group, "A Phase III Comparative Study of Three Non-Nucleoside Reverse Transcriptase Inhibitor (NNRTI) Sparing Antiretroviral Regimens for Treatment-Naïve

T. Sozu et al., *Sample Size Determination in Clinical Trials with Multiple Endpoints*, SpringerBriefs in Statistics, DOI 10.1007/978-3-319-22005-5_1

HIV-1-Infected Volunteers (The ARDENT Study: Atazanavir, Raltegravir, or Darunavir with Emtricitabine/Tenofovir for Naïve Treatment)" is designed with two co-primary endpoints: time to virologic failure (efficacy endpoint) and time to discontinuation of randomized treatment due to toxicity (safety endpoint). Coinfection/comorbidity studies may utilize co-primary endpoints to evaluate multiple comorbities, e.g., a trial evaluating therapies to treat Kaposi's sarcoma (KS) in HIV-infected individuals may have the time to KS progression and the time to HIV virologic failure, as co-primary endpoints. Infectious disease trials may use time-to-clinical-cure and time-to-microbiological cure as co-primary endpoints. Trials evaluating strategies to decrease antimicrobial use may use clinical outcome and antimicrobial use as co-primary endpoints.

Regulators have also issued guidelines recommending co-primary endpoints in specific disease areas. The Committee for Medicinal Products for Human Use (CHMP) issued a guideline (2008) recommending the use of cognitive, functional, and global endpoints to evaluate symptomatic improvement of dementia associated with in Alzheimer's disease, indicating that primary endpoints should be stipulated reflecting the cognitive and functional disease components. In the design of clinical trials evaluating treatments in patients affected by irritable bowel syndrome (IBS), the U.S. Food and Drug Administration (FDA) recommends the use of two endpoints for assessing IBS signs and symptoms: (1) pain intensity and stool frequency of IBS with constipation (IBS-C), and (2) pain intensity and stool consistency of IBS with diarrhea (IBS-D) (Food and Drug Administration 2012). CHMP (2012) also discusses the use of two endpoints for assessing IBS signs and symptoms, i.e., global assessment of symptoms and assessment of symptoms of abdominal discomfort/pain, but they are different from FDA's recommendation. Offen et al. (2007) provides other examples.

The resulting need for new approaches to the design and analysis of clinical trials has been noted (Dmitrienko et al. 2010; Gong et al. 2000; Hung and Wang 2009; Offen et al. 2007). Utilizing multiple endpoints may provide the opportunity for characterizing intervention's multidimensional effects, but also creates challenges. Specifically controlling type I and type II error rates is non-trivial when the multiple primary endpoints are potentially correlated. When more than one endpoint is viewed as important in a clinical trial, then a decision must be made as to whether it is desirable to evaluate the joint effects on ALL endpoints or AT LEAST ONE of the endpoints. This decision defines the alternative hypothesis to be tested and provides a framework for approaching trial design. When designing the trial to evaluate the joint effects on ALL of the endpoints, no adjustment is needed to control the type I error rate. The hypothesis associated with each endpoint can be evaluated at the same significance level that is desired for demonstrating effects on all of the endpoints (ICH-E9 Guideline 1998). However, the type II error rate increases as the number of endpoints to be evaluated increases. This is referred to as "multiple co-primary endpoints" and is related to the intersection-union problem (Hung and Wang 2009; Offen et al. 2007). In contrast, when designing the trial to evaluate an effect on AT LEAST ONE of the endpoints, then an adjustment is needed to control the type I error rate. This is referred to as "multiple primary endpoints" or "alternative

Table 1.1 Summary of references discussing sample size methods in clinical trials with multiple endpoints

Endpoint scale	Alternative hypothesis	
	Effect on all endpoints	Effect on at least one endpoint
Continuous	Chuang-Stein et al. (2007)	Dmitrienko et al. (2010)
	Dmitrienko et al. (2010)	Gong et al. (2000)
	Eaton and Muirhead (2007)	Hung and Wang (2009)
	Hung and Wang (2009)	Senn and Bretz (2007)
	Julious and McIntyre (2012)	
	Kordzakhia et al. (2010)	
	Offen et al. (2007)	
	Senn and Bretz (2007)	
	Sozu et al. (2006, 2011)	
	Sugimoto et al. (2012a)	
	Xiong et al. (2005)	
Binary	Hamasaki et al. (2012)	Hamasaki et al. (2012)
	Song (2009)	
	Sozu et al. (2010, 2011)	
Time-to-event	Hamasaki et al. (2013)	Sugimoto et al. (2012b)
	Sugimoto et al. (2011, 2012b, 2013)	
Mixed	Sozu et al. (2012)	Sugimoto et al. (2012b)
	Sugimoto et al. (2012b)	

primary endpoints" (Offen et al. 2007) and is related to the union-intersection problem (Dmitrienko et al. 2010).

In such clinical trials, the correlation among the multiple endpoints should be considered in order to obtain an appropriate sample size. However the correlation is usually unknown and thus must be estimated with external data. One potential alternative to multiple endpoints is to define a single composite endpoint based on the multiple endpoints. This effectively reduces the problem to a single dimension and thus simplifies the design to avoid the multiplicity issues regarding multiple endpoints. However the creation and interpretation of a composite endpoint can be challenging particularly when treatments effects vary across components with very different clinical importance (Cordoba et al. 2010). As summarized in Table 1.1, several methods for power and sample size calculations have proposed for clinical trials with multiple endpoints that consider the correlations among the endpoints into the calculations.

Continuous endpoints: Xiong et al. (2005) discussed overall power and sample size for clinical trials with two co-primary continuous endpoints assuming that the two endpoints are bivariate normally distributed and their variance-covariance matrix is known. Sozu et al. (2006) extended their method to continuous endpoints assuming that the variance-covariance matrix is unknown using the Wishart distribution. Sozu et al. (2011) discussed extensions to more than two continuous endpoints for both known and unknown variances. Sugimoto et al. (2012a) discussed a convenient and practical formula for sample size calculation with multiple continuous endpoints. Eaton and Muirhead (2007) discussed the properties of the testing procedure including testing each endpoint separately at the same significance level using two-sample t-tests, and rejecting only if each t-statistic is significant. They showed that the test may be conservative and that it is biased. In addition, they provided a simple expression for calculating the p-value and computable bounds for the overall power function. Julious and McIntyre (2012) summarized three methods of sample size calculation in the framework of clinical trials involving multiple comparisons. Since the testing procedure for co-primary endpoints may be conservative, the methods can result in large and impractical sample sizes. To address this problem, Patel (1991), Chuang-Stein et al. (2007) and Kordzakhia et al. (2010) discussed methods to control the type I error rate. The methods may lead to relatively smaller sample sizes, but may also introduce other issues.

Binary endpoints: Sozu et al. (2010, 2011) discussed the overall power and sample size calculations in superiority clinical trials with co-primary binary endpoints assuming that the binary endpoints are jointly distributed as a multivariate Bernoulli distribution. They noted notable practical and technical issues during estimation of the correlation due to the higher number of endpoints imposing important restrictions on the correlation. Hamasaki et al. (2012) provided the sample size calculations for trials using with multiple risk ratios and odds ratios as primary contrasts. Song (2009) discussed sample size calculations with co-primary binary endpoints in non-inferiority clinical trials, but did not discuss such a restriction on the correlation.

During the last several years, our team has conducted extensive research on sample size determination in clinical trials with multiple endpoints. This book summarizes our results in an integrated manner to help biostatisticians involved in clinical trials to understand the appropriate sample size methodologies. The focus of the book is aimed at power and sample size determination for comparing the effect of two interventions in superiority clinical trials with multiple endpoints. We focus on discussing the methods for sample size calculation in clinical trials when the alternative hypothesis is that there are effects on ALL endpoints. We only briefly discuss trials designed with an alternative hypothesis of an effect on AT LEAST ONE endpoint with a prespecified non-ordering of endpoints. The structure of the book is as follows:

Chapter 2 provides an overview of the concepts and technical fundamentals regarding power and sample size calculation for clinical trials with multiple continuous co-primary endpoints. Numerical examples illustrate the methods. The chapter also introduces conservative sample sizing strategies.

Chapter 3 provides methods for power and sample size determination for clinical trials with multiple co-primary binary endpoints. The chapter introduces the three correlation structures defining the association among the endpoints and discusses the overall power and sample size calculation for five methods: the one-sided chi-square test with and without the continuity correction, the arcsine root transformation method with and without the continuity correction, and the Fisher's exact test.

The methods discussed in Chaps. 2 and 3 require considerable mathematical sophistication and programming. To improve the practical utility of these methods, Chap. 4 describes a more efficient and practical algorithm for calculating the sample sizes and presents a useful sample size formula with numerical tables. An example demonstrating how to use the sample size formula and numerical tables is provided. Codes in R and SAS software packages are described and available in the Appendix.

Chapter 5 provides an overview of the concepts and technical fundamentals regarding power and sample size determination for clinical trials with multiple continuous primary endpoints, i.e., when the alternative hypothesis is that there are effects on at least one endpoint.

Our work to date has been restricted to (i) continuous and (ii) binary endpoints in a superiority clinical trial with two interventions. However, this work provides a foundation for designing randomized trials with other design features including non-inferiority clinical trials, clinical trials with more than two interventions, trials with time-to-event endpoints or mixed-scale endpoints, and group sequential clinical trials. Chapter 6 briefly mentions how our results may be extended to design such trials.

References

Chuang-Stein C, Stryszak P, Dmitrienko A, Offen W (2007) Challenge of multiple co-primary endpoints: a new approach. Stat Med 26:1181–1192

Committee for Medicinal Products for Human Use (CHMP). Concept paper on the revision of the CHMP points to consider on the evaluation of medicinal products for the treatment of irritable bowel syndrome (CPMP/EWP/785/97) (EMA/CHMP/172616/2012). EMA: London, 2012. http://www.ema.europa.eu/docs/en_GB/document_library/Scientific_guideline/2012/06/WC500128217.pdf Accessed 9 June 2014

Cordoba G, Schwartz L, Woloshin S, Bae H, Gotzsche PC (2010) Definition, reporting, and interpretation of composite outcomes in clinical trials: systematic review. Br Med J 341:c3920

Dmitrienko A, Tamhane AC, Bretz F (2010) Multiple testing problems in pharmaceutical statistics. Chapman & Hall/CRC, Boca Raton

Eaton ML, Muirhead RJ (2007) On a multiple endpoints testing problem. J Stat Plan Infer 137:3416–3429

Food and Drug Administration (FDA). Guidance for industry irritable bowel syndrome—clinical evaluation of drugs for treatment. Center for Drug Evaluation and Research, Food and Drug Administration, Silver Spring, MD, 2012. http://www.fda.gov/downloads/Drugs/Guidances/UCM205269.pdf Accessed 9 June 2014

Gong J, Pinheiro JC, DeMets DL (2000) Estimating significance level and power comparisons for testing multiple endpoints in clinical trials. Control Clin Trials 21:323–329

Hamasaki T, Sugimoto T, Evans SR, Sozu T (2013) Sample size determination for clinical trials with co-primary outcomes: exponential event-times. Pharma Stat 12:28–34

Hamasaki T, Evans SR, Sugimoto T, Sozu T (2012) Power and sample size determination for clinical trials with two correlated binary relative risks. In: ENAR Spring Meeting 2012; 2012 April 1–4; Washington DC, USA

Hung HM, Wang SJ (2009) Some controversial multiple testing problems in regulatory applications. J Biopharm Stat 19:1–11

International conference on harmonisation of technical requirements for registration of pharmaceuticals for human use. ICH tripartite guideline. Statistical principles for clinical trials. 1998. http://www.ich.org/fileadmin/Public_Web_Site/ICH_Products/Guidelines/Efficacy/E9/Step4/E9_Guideline.pdf Accessed 9 June 2014

Julious SA, McIntyre NE (2012) Sample sizes for trials involving multiple correlated must-win comparisons. Pharm Stat 11:177–185

Kordzakhia G, Siddiqui O, Huque MF (2010) Method of balanced adjustment in testing co-primary endpoints. Stat Med 29:2055–2066

Offen W, Chuang-Stein C, Dmitrienko A, Littman G, Maca J, Meyerson L, Muirhead R, Stryszak P, Boddy A, Chen K, Copley-Merriman K, Dere W, Givens S, Hall D, Henry D, Jackson JD, Krishen A, Liu T, Ryder S, Sankoh AJ, Wang J, Yeh CH (2007) Multiple co-primary endpoints: medical and statistical solutions. Drug Inf J 41:31–46

Patel HI (1991) Comparison of treatments in a combination therapy trial. J Biopharm Stat 1:171–183

Senn S, Bretz F (2007) Power and sample size when multiple endpoints are considered. Pharm Stat 6:161–170

Song JX (2009) Sample size for simultaneous testing of rate differences in noninferiority trials with multiple endpoints. Comput Stat Data Anal 53:1201–1207

Sozu T, Kanou T, Hamada C, Yoshimura I (2006) Power and sample size calculations in clinical trials with multiple primary variables. Japan J Biometrics 27:83–96

Sozu T, Sugimoto T, Hamasaki T (2010) Sample size determination in clinical trials with multiple co-primary binary endpoints. Stat Med 29:2169–2179

Sozu T, Sugimoto T, Hamasaki T (2011) Sample size determination in superiority clinical trials with multiple co-primary correlated endpoints. J Biopharm Stat 21:650–668

Sozu T, Sugimoto T, Hamasaki T (2012) Sample size determination in clinical trials with multiple co-primary endpoints including mixed continuous and binary variables. Biometrical J 54:716–729

Sugimoto T, Hamasaki T, Sozu T (2011) Sample size determination in clinical trials with two correlated co-primary time-to-event endpoints. In: The 7th international conference on multiple comparison procedures, Washington DC, USA, 29 Aug–1 Sept

Sugimoto T, Sozu T, Hamasaki T (2012a) A convenient formula for sample size calculations in clinical trials with multiple co-primary continuous endpoints. Pharm Stat 11:118–128

Sugimoto T, Hamasaki T, Sozu T, Evans SR (2012b) Sample size determination in clinical trials with two correlated time-to-event endpoints as primary contrast. In: The 6th FDA-DIA statistics forum, Washington DC, USA, 22–25 April

Sugimoto T, Sozu T, Hamasaki T, Evans SR (2013) A logrank test-based method for sizing clinical trials with two co-primary time-to-events endpoints. Biostatistics 14:409–421

Xiong C, Yu K, Gao F, Yan Y, Zhang Z (2005) Power and sample size for clinical trials when efficacy is required in multiple endpoints: application to an Alzheimer's treatment trial. Clin Trials 2:387–393

Chapter 2
Continuous Co-primary Endpoints

Abstract In this chapter, we provide an overview of the concepts and the technical fundamentals regarding power and sample size calculation when comparing two interventions with multiple co-primary continuous endpoints in a clinical trial. We provide numerical examples to illustrate the methods and introduce conservative sample sizing strategies for these clinical trials.

Keywords Conjunctive power · Conservative sample size · Intersection-union test · Multivariate normal

2.1 Introduction

Consider a randomized clinical trial comparing two interventions with n_T subjects in the test group and n_C subjects in the control group. There are $K (\geq 2)$ co-primary continuous endpoints with a K-variate normal distribution. Let the responses for the n_T subjects in the test group be denoted by Y_{Tjk}, $j = 1, \ldots, n_T$, and those for the n_C subjects in the control group, by Y_{Cjk}, $j = 1, \ldots, n_C$. Suppose that the vectors of responses $Y_{Tj} = (Y_{Tj1}, \ldots, Y_{TjK})^T$ and $Y_{Cj} = (Y_{Cj1}, \ldots, Y_{CjK})^T$ are independently distributed as K-variate normal distributions with mean vectors $E[Y_{Tj}] = \mu_T = (\mu_{T1}, \ldots, \mu_{TK})^T$ and $E[Y_{Cj}] = \mu_C = (\mu_{C1}, \ldots, \mu_{CK})^T$, respectively, and common covariance matrix Σ, i.e.,

$$Y_{Tj} \sim N_K(\mu_T, \Sigma) \quad \text{and} \quad Y_{Cj} \sim N_K(\mu_C, \Sigma),$$

where

$$\Sigma = \begin{pmatrix} \sigma_1^2 & \cdots & \rho^{1K}\sigma_1\sigma_K \\ \vdots & \ddots & \vdots \\ \rho^{1K}\sigma_1\sigma_K & \cdots & \sigma_K^2 \end{pmatrix}$$

with $\text{var}[Y_{Tjk}] = \text{var}[Y_{Cjk}] = \sigma_k^2$, $\text{corr}[Y_{Tjk}, Y_{Tjk'}] = \text{corr}[Y_{Cjk}, Y_{Cjk'}] = \rho^{kk'}$ $(k \neq k' : 1 \leq k < k' \leq K)$. In this setting, $\rho^{kk'}$ is the association measure among the endpoints.

© The Author(s) 2015

T. Sozu et al., *Sample Size Determination in Clinical Trials with Multiple Endpoints*, SpringerBriefs in Statistics, DOI 10.1007/978-3-319-22005-5_2

We are interested in estimating the difference in the means $\mu_{Tk} - \mu_{Ck}$. A positive value of $\mu_{Tk} - \mu_{Ck}$ indicates an intervention benefit. We assert the superiority of the test intervention over the control in terms of all K primary endpoints if and only if $\mu_{Tk} - \mu_{Ck} > 0$ for all $k = 1, \ldots, K$. Thus, the hypotheses for testing are

$$H_0 : \mu_{Tk} - \mu_{Ck} \leq 0 \text{ for at least one } k,$$
$$H_1 : \mu_{Tk} - \mu_{Ck} > 0 \text{ for all } k.$$

In testing the preceding hypotheses, the null hypothesis H_0 is rejected if and only if all of the null hypotheses associated with each of the K primary endpoints are rejected at a significance level of α. The corresponding rejection region is the intersection of K regions associated with the K co-primary endpoints; therefore the test used in data analysis is an intersection-union test (IUT) (Berger 1982).

2.2 Test Statistics and Power

2.2.1 Known Variance

Assume that σ_k^2 is known. The following Z-statistic can be used to test the difference in the means for each endpoint:

$$Z_k = \frac{\bar{Y}_{Tk} - \bar{Y}_{Ck}}{\sigma_k \sqrt{\dfrac{1}{n_T} + \dfrac{1}{n_C}}}, \quad k = 1, \ldots, K, \tag{2.1}$$

where $\bar{Y}_{Tk}$ and $\bar{Y}_{Ck}$ are the sample means given by

$$\bar{Y}_{Tk} = \frac{1}{n_T} \sum_{j=1}^{n_T} Y_{Tjk} \quad \text{and} \quad \bar{Y}_{Ck} = \frac{1}{n_C} \sum_{j=1}^{n_C} Y_{Cjk}.$$

The overall power function for the Z-statistics in (2.1) can be written as

$$1 - \beta = \Pr\left[\bigcap_{k=1}^{K} \{Z_k > z_\alpha\} \,\middle|\, H_1 \right] = \Pr\left[\bigcap_{k=1}^{K} \{Z_k^* > c_k^*\} \,\middle|\, H_1 \right], \tag{2.2}$$

where $Z_k^* = Z_k - \sqrt{\kappa n}\delta_k$, $c_k^* = z_\alpha - \sqrt{\kappa n}\delta_k$, $\delta_k = (\mu_{Tk} - \mu_{Ck})/\sigma_k$ (standardized effect size), $r = n_C/n_T$, $n = n_T$, and $\kappa = r/(1 + r)$. Further, z_α is the $(1 - \alpha)$ quantile of the standard normal distribution. This overall power (2.2) is referred to as "complete power" (Westfall et al. 2011) or "conjunctive power" (Bretz et al. 2011; Senn and Bretz 2007). Since $E[Z_k^*] = 0$ and $var[Z_k^*] = 1$, the vector of $(Z_1^*, \ldots, Z_K^*)^T$ is distributed as a K-variate normal distribution, $N_K(\mathbf{0}, \rho_Z)$, where the off-diagonal element of $\boldsymbol{\rho}_Z$ is given by $\rho^{kk'}$. The overall power function is calculated using $\Phi_K(-c_1^*, \ldots, -c_K^*)$, where Φ_K is the cumulative distribution function of $N_K(\mathbf{0}, \boldsymbol{\rho}_Z)$.

2.2.2 Unknown Variance

We assume that σ_k^2 is unknown as is realistic in practice. The following T-statistic can be used to test the difference in the means for each endpoint:

$$T_k = \frac{\bar{Y}_{Tk} - \bar{Y}_{Ck}}{s_k \sqrt{\dfrac{1}{n_T} + \dfrac{1}{n_C}}}, \quad k = 1, \ldots, K, \tag{2.3}$$

where $\bar{Y}_{Tk}$ and $\bar{Y}_{Ck}$ are the sample means defined in the previous section, and s_k is the usual pooled standard deviation given by

$$s_k^2 = \frac{\sum_{j=1}^{n_T}(Y_{Tjk} - \bar{Y}_{Tk})^2 + \sum_{j=1}^{n_C}(Y_{Cjk} - \bar{Y}_{Ck})^2}{n_T + n_C - 2}.$$

Let $\boldsymbol{D} = (D_1, \ldots, D_K)^T$ with $D_k = (\bar{Y}_{Tk} - \bar{Y}_{Ck})/\sigma_k$, then $\sqrt{\kappa n}\boldsymbol{D}$ is distributed as a K-variate normal distribution with mean vector $\sqrt{\kappa n}\boldsymbol{\delta}$ and covariance matrix $\boldsymbol{\rho}_Z$, namely, $N_K(\sqrt{\kappa n}\boldsymbol{\delta}, \boldsymbol{\rho}_Z)$. In addition, the pooled matrix of the sums of squares and cross products,

$$\boldsymbol{W} = \begin{pmatrix} w_{11} & \cdots & w_{1K} \\ \vdots & \ddots & \vdots \\ w_{1K} & \cdots & w_{KK} \end{pmatrix}$$

is distributed as a Wishart distribution with $n_T + n_C - 2$ degree of freedom and covariance matrix $\boldsymbol{\rho}_Z$ where

$$w_{kk'} = \begin{cases} \dfrac{1}{\sigma_k^2}\left(\displaystyle\sum_{j=1}^{n_T}(Y_{Tjk} - \bar{Y}_{Tk})^2 + \sum_{j=1}^{n_C}(Y_{Cjk} - \bar{Y}_{Ck})^2\right), & k = k', \\[3ex] \dfrac{1}{\sigma_k\sigma_{k'}}\left(\displaystyle\sum_{j=1}^{n_T}(Y_{Tjk} - \bar{Y}_{Tk})(Y_{Tjk'} - \bar{Y}_{Tk'}) + \sum_{j=1}^{n_C}(Y_{Cjk} - \bar{Y}_{Ck})(Y_{Cjk'} - \bar{Y}_{Ck'})\right), & k \neq k'. \end{cases}$$

Please see, e.g., Johnson and Kotz (1972) for the definition of the Wishart distribution. Subsequently statistic (2.3) can be rewritten as

$$T_k = \frac{\sqrt{\kappa n}D_k}{\sqrt{\dfrac{w_{kk}}{n_T + n_C - 2}}}$$

and the overall power function for statistic (2.3) is given by

$$1 - \beta = \Pr\left[\bigcap_{k=1}^{K} \{T_k > t_{\alpha,n_T+n_C-2}\} \,\middle|\, H_1\right],\tag{2.4}$$

where t_{α,n_T+n_C-2} is the $(1-\alpha)$ quantile of the t-distribution with n_T+n_C-2 degrees of freedom. If $K = 1$, then the overall power function (2.4) is based on a noncentral univariate t-distribution (e.g., Julious 2009). If $K \geq 2$, then the joint distribution of T_k is not a multivariate noncentral t-distribution because the joint distribution of $w_{kk'}$ is a Wishart distribution, which is not included in a multivariate gamma distribution. Hence, in order to calculate the overall power function of such a distribution, we consider rewriting (2.4) as

$$\begin{aligned}
1 - \beta &= \Pr\left[\bigcap_{k=1}^{K} \left\{\sqrt{\kappa n}D_k > t_{\alpha,n_T+n_C-2}\sqrt{\frac{w_{kk}}{n_T+n_C-2}}\right\} \,\middle|\, H_1\right] \\
&= \mathrm{E}\left[\Pr\left[\bigcap_{k=1}^{K} \{Z_k^* > c_k^*(w_{kk})\} \,\middle|\, W\right]\right] \\
&= \mathrm{E}\left[\Phi_K(-c_1^*(w_{11}),\ldots,-c_K^*(w_{KK}))\right],
\end{aligned}\tag{2.5}$$

where

$$c_k^*(w_{kk}) = t_{\alpha,n_T+n_C-2}\sqrt{\frac{w_{kk}}{n_T+n_C-2}} - \sqrt{\kappa n}\delta_k \quad (\delta_k > 0 \text{ for all } k).$$

The equation (2.5) is calculated by a simulated average of $\Phi_K(-c_1^*(w_{11}),\ldots,-c_K^*(w_{KK}))$ obtained by generating random numbers of W. For additional details, please see Sozu et al. (2006).

2.3 Sample Size Calculation

In the sample size calculation, the means μ_{Tk}, μ_{Ck}, the variance σ_k^2, and the correlation coefficient $\rho^{kk'}$ must be specified in advance. The sample size required to achieve the desired overall power of $1-\beta$ at the significance level of α is the smallest integer not less than n satisfying $1 - \beta \leq \Phi_K(-c_1^*,\ldots,-c_K^*)$ for the known variance and $1 - \beta \leq \mathrm{E}\left[\Phi_K(-c_1^*(w_{11}),\ldots,-c_K^*(w_{KK}))\right]$ for the unknown variance. An iterative procedure is required to find the required sample size. The easiest way is a grid search to increase n gradually until the power under n exceeds the desired overall power of $1-\beta$, where the maximum value of the sample sizes separately calculated for each endpoint can be used as the initial value for sample size calculation. However, this often takes much computing time. To improve the convenience in the sample size calculation, Chap. 4 provides a more efficient and practical algorithm for calculating the sample sizes and presents a useful sample size formula with numerical tables for multiple co-primary endpoints.

When the standardized effect size for one endpoint is relatively smaller than that for other endpoints, then the sample size is determined by the smallest standardized effect size and does not greatly depend on the correlation. In this situation, the sample size equation for co-primary continuous endpoints can be simplified, using the equation for the singe continuous endpoint, as given by Eq. (2.8) in Sect. 2.5.

2.4 Behavior of the Type I Error Rate, Power and Sample Size

We focus on the behavior of the type I error rate, overall power and sample size calculated using the method based on the known variance in Sect. 2.2.1, because the method based on the unknown variance in Sect. 2.2.2 provides similar results. Sozu et al. (2011) show that the sample size per group calculated using the method based on the unknown variance is generally one participant larger than that using the method based on the known variance.

2.4.1 Type I Error Rate

There are alternative hypotheses in which the corresponding powers are lower than the nominal significance level in order to keep the maximum type I error rate below the nominal significance level as described in the ICH (1998). For more details, please see Chuang-Stein et al. (2007) and Eaton and Muirhead (2007).

Figure 2.1 illustrates the behavior of type I error rate for $\alpha = 0.025$ as a function of the correlation, where the off-diagonal elements of the correlation matrix are equal, i.e., $\rho = \rho^{12} = \cdots = \rho^{K-1,K}$, and all of the standardized effect sizes are zero, i.e., $\delta_1 = \cdots = \delta_K = 0$ ($K = 2, 3, 4, 5,$ and 10).

Fig. 2.1 Behavior of the type I error rate as a function of the correlation, where the off-diagonal elements of the correlation matrix are equal, i.e., $\rho = \rho^{12} = \cdots = \rho^{K-1,K}$, and all of the standardized effect sizes are zero, i.e., $\delta_1 = \cdots = \delta_K = 0$

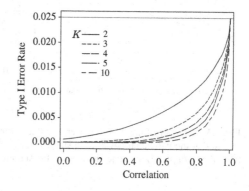

Fig. 2.2 Behavior of the
type I error rate as a function
of the correlation when there
are two co-primary
endpoints ($K = 2$)

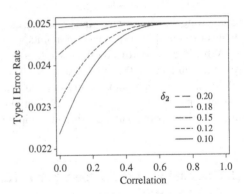

Figure 2.2 illustrates the behavior of type I error rate for $\alpha = 0.025$ as a function
of the correlation when there are two co-primary endpoints ($K = 2$), where $\delta_1 = 0$
and $\delta_2 = 0.10, 0.12, 0.15, 0.18$, and 2.0.

2.4.2 Overall Power

Figure 2.3 illustrates the behavior of overall power $1 - \beta$ as a function of the correlation for a given equal sample size per group $n = n_T = n_C$ (i.e., $r = 1.0$) so
that the individual power for a single primary endpoint is at least 0.80 and 0.90 by a
one-sided test at the significance level of $\alpha = 0.025$. Here, the off-diagonal elements
of the correlation matrix are equal, i.e., $\rho = \rho^{12} = \cdots = \rho^{K-1,K}$, and all of the
standardized effect sizes are equal to 0.2, i.e., $\delta_1 = \cdots = \delta_K = 0.2$ ($K = 2, 3, 4, 5$,
and 10). The figure illustrates that the overall power increases as the correlation
approaches one and decreases as the number of endpoints to be evaluated increases.

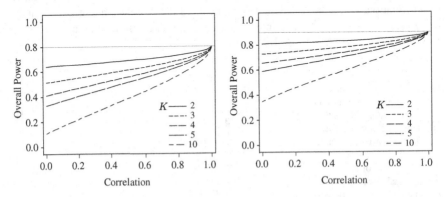

Fig. 2.3 Behavior of the overall power $1 - \beta$ as a function of the correlation for a given sample
size so that the individual power for a single primary endpoint is at least 0.80 (the *left panel*) and
0.90 (the *right panel*) by a one-sided test at the significance level of $\alpha = 0.025$

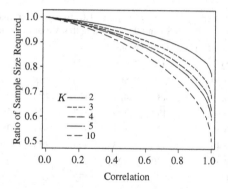

Fig. 2.4 Behavior of the ratio $(n(\rho)/n(0))$ as a function of the correlation, where the off-diagonal elements of the correlation matrix are equal, i.e., $\rho = \rho^{12} = \cdots = \rho^{K-1,K}$, and all of the standardized effect sizes are equal to 0.2, i.e., $\delta_1 = \cdots = \delta_K = 0.2$ ($K = 2, 3, 4, 5$, and 10). The sample size was calculated with the overall power of $1 - \beta = 0.80$ when each of the K endpoints is tested at the significance level of $\alpha = 0.025$ by a one-sided test

2.4.3 Sample Size

Figure 2.4 illustrates the behavior of the ratio of $n(\rho)$ to $n(0)$ as a function of the correlation when there are K co-primary endpoints ($K = 2, 3, 4, 5$, and 10), where the off-diagonal elements of the correlation matrix are equal $\rho = \rho^{12} = \cdots = \rho^{K-1,K}$, and all of the standardized effect sizes are equal to 0.2, i.e., $\delta_1 = \cdots = \delta_K = 0.2$. The equal sample sizes per group $n = n_T = n_C$ (i.e., $r = 1.0$) were calculated with the overall power of $1 - \beta = 0.80$ when each of the K endpoints is tested at the significance level of $\alpha = 0.025$ by a one-sided test. The figure illustrates that the ratio $n(\rho)/n(0)$ becomes smaller as the correlation approaches one and the degree of reduction is larger as the number of endpoints to be evaluated increases.

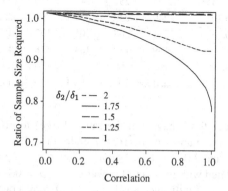

Fig. 2.5 Behavior of the ratio $(n(\rho)/n(0))$ as a function of the correlation for two co-primary endpoints ($K = 2$). The sample size was calculated with the overall power of $1 - \beta = 0.80$ when each of the two endpoints is tested at the significance level of $\alpha = 0.025$ by a one-sided test

Table 2.1 Sample size per group ($n = n_T = n_C, r = 1.0$) for two co-primary endpoints ($K = 2$) with the overall power of $1 - \beta = 0.80$ and 0.9 assuming that variance is known

Targeted power	Standardized effect size δ_1	δ_2	Correlation ρ^{12} 0.0	0.3	0.5	0.8	1.0	E_1	E_2
0.80	0.20	0.20	516	503	490	458	393	393	393
	0.20	0.25	432	424	417	401	393	393	252
	0.20	0.30	402	399	397	393	393	393	175
	0.20	0.35	394	394	393	393	393	393	129
	0.20	0.40	393	393	393	393	393	393	99
	0.25	0.25	330	322	314	294	252	252	252
	0.25	0.30	284	278	272	260	252	252	175
	0.25	0.35	263	260	257	253	252	252	129
	0.25	0.40	254	253	253	252	252	252	99
	0.30	0.30	230	224	218	204	175	175	175
	0.30	0.35	201	197	192	183	175	175	129
	0.30	0.40	186	183	181	176	175	175	99
	0.35	0.35	169	165	160	150	129	129	129
	0.35	0.40	150	147	143	136	129	129	99
	0.40	0.40	129	126	123	115	99	99	99
0.90	0.20	0.20	646	637	626	597	526	526	526
	0.20	0.25	552	547	542	531	526	526	337
	0.20	0.30	529	528	527	526	526	526	234
	0.20	0.35	526	526	526	526	526	526	172
	0.20	0.40	526	526	526	526	526	526	132
	0.25	0.25	413	408	401	382	337	337	337
	0.25	0.30	360	356	352	343	337	337	234
	0.25	0.35	342	340	339	337	337	337	172
	0.25	0.40	337	337	337	337	337	337	132
	0.30	0.30	287	283	279	265	234	234	234
	0.30	0.35	254	251	248	240	234	234	172
	0.30	0.40	240	239	237	235	234	234	132
	0.35	0.35	211	208	205	195	172	172	172
	0.35	0.40	189	187	184	178	172	172	132
	0.40	0.40	162	160	157	150	132	132	132

E_1, E_2: Sample size separately calculated for each endpoint 1 and 2 so that the individual power is at least 0.8 and 0.9

Figure 2.5 illustrates the behavior of the ratio of $n(\rho)$ to $n(0)$ as a function of the correlation when there are two co-primary endpoints ($K = 2$), where $\delta_2/\delta_1 = 1.0, 1.25, 1.50, 1.75$, and 2.0. The equal sample sizes per group $n = n_T = n_C$ (i.e., $r = 1.0$) were calculated with the overall power of $1 - \beta = 0.80$ when each of two endpoints is tested at the significance level of $\alpha = 0.025$ by a one-sided test and the vertical axis is the ratio of $n(\rho^{12})$ to $n(0)$. When $\delta_2/\delta_1 = 1.0$, the ratio ($n(\rho)/n(0)$) decreases as the correlation approaches one. Even when $1.0 < \delta_2/\delta_1 < 1.5$, the ratio

Table 2.2 Sample size per group ($n = n_T = n_C, r = 1.0$) for three endpoints ($K = 3$) with the overall power of $1 - \beta = 0.80$ and 0.9 assuming that variance is known

| Targeted power | Standardized effect size | | | Correlation ρ^{12} | | | | | | | |
	δ_1	δ_2	δ_3	0.0	0.3	0.5	0.8	1.0	E_1	E_2	E_3
0.80	0.20	0.20	0.20	586	566	545	494	393	393	393	393
	0.20	0.20	0.30	517	504	490	458	393	393	393	175
	0.20	0.20	0.40	516	503	490	458	393	393	393	099
	0.20	0.30	0.30	410	404	400	394	393	393	175	175
	0.20	0.30	0.40	402	399	397	393	393	393	175	99
	0.20	0.40	0.40	393	393	393	393	393	393	99	99
	0.30	0.30	0.30	261	252	242	220	175	175	175	175
	0.30	0.30	0.40	233	226	220	204	175	175	175	99
	0.30	0.40	0.40	194	190	186	177	175	175	99	99
	0.40	0.40	0.40	147	142	137	124	99	99	99	99
0.90	0.20	0.20	0.20	714	700	683	635	526	526	526	526
	0.20	0.20	0.30	646	637	626	597	526	526	526	234
	0.20	0.20	0.40	646	637	626	597	526	526	526	132
	0.20	0.30	0.30	532	530	528	526	526	526	234	234
	0.20	0.30	0.40	529	528	527	526	526	526	234	132
	0.20	0.40	0.40	526	526	526	526	526	526	132	132
	0.30	0.30	0.30	318	311	304	283	234	234	234	234
	0.30	0.30	0.40	289	284	279	266	234	234	234	132
	0.30	0.40	0.40	245	243	240	235	234	234	132	132
	0.40	0.40	0.40	179	175	171	159	132	132	132	132

E_1, E_2, E_3: Sample size separately calculated for each endpoint 1, 2, and 3 so that the individual power is at least 0.8 and 0.9

($n(\rho)/n(0)$) still decreases as the correlation approaches one. However, when the ratio δ_2/δ_1 exceeds 1.5, the ratio ($n(\rho)/n(0)$) does not change considerably as the correlation varies.

Table 2.1 provides the equal sample sizes per group ($n = n_T = n_C, r = 1.0$) for two co-primary endpoints ($K = 2$) with correlation $\rho^{12} = 0.0$ (no correlation), 0.3 (low correlation), 0.5 (moderate correlation), 0.8 (high correlation), and 1.0 (perfect correlation). The sample size was calculated to detect standardized effect sizes of $0.2 \leq \delta_1, \delta_2 \leq 0.4$ with the overall power of $1 - \beta = 0.80$, when each of the two endpoints is tested at the significance level of $\alpha = 0.025$ by a one-sided test.

In the cases of equal effect sizes between the two endpoints, that is, $\delta_1 = \delta_2$, the sample size decreases as the correlation approaches one. Comparing the cases of $\rho^{12} = 0.0$ and $\rho^{12} = 0.8$, the decrease in the sample size is approximately 11 %. Even in the cases of unequal effect sizes, that is, $\delta_1 < \delta_2$, the sample sizes decrease as the correlation approaches one. However, when the ratio δ_2/δ_1 exceeds roughly 1.5, the sample size does not change considerably as the correlation varies. Consequently, the sample size is determined by the smaller effect size and is approximately equal to that calculated on the basis of the smaller effect size.

Similar to the case of two endpoints, Table 2.2 provides the equal sample sizes per group for three endpoints ($K = 3$) to detect standardized effect sizes $0.2 \leq \delta_1, \delta_2, \delta_3 \leq 0.4$ with overall power $1 - \beta = 0.8$ when each of the three endpoints is tested at the significance level of $\alpha = 0.025$ by a one-sided test, where the off-diagonal elements of the correlation matrix are equal, i.e., $\rho = \rho^{12} = \rho^{13} = \rho^{23} = 0.0, 0.3, 0.5, 0.8$, and 1.0. In the cases of equal effect sizes among three endpoints, that is, $\delta_1 = \delta_2 = \delta_3$, the sample size decreases as the correlation approaches one. For example, comparing the cases of $\rho = 0.0$ and $\rho = 0.8$, the decrease in the sample size is approximately 16%. Even in the cases of unequal effect sizes, that is, $\delta_1 < \delta_2 \leq \delta_3$, the sample size decreases as the correlation approaches one. However, when the ratios δ_2/δ_1 and δ_3/δ_1 exceed 1.5, the sample size does not change as the correlation varies. Consequently, the sample size is determined by the smallest effect size and is approximately equal to that calculated on the basis of the smallest effect size.

2.5 Conservative Sample Size Determination

When clinical trialists face the challenge of sizing clinical trials with multiple endpoints, one major concern is whether the correlations among the endpoints should be considered in the sample size calculation. The correlations may be estimated from external or internal pilot data, but they are usually unknown. When there are more than two endpoints, estimating the correlations is extremely difficult. If the correlations are over-estimated and are included into the sample size calculation for evaluating the joint effects on all of the endpoints, then the sample size is too small and important effects may not be detected. As a conservative approach, one could assume zero correlations among the endpoints as the overall power for detecting the joint statistical significance is lowest when the correlation is zero for $\rho^{kk'} \geq 0$.

Consider a conservative sample size strategy when evaluating superiority for ALL continuous endpoints by using a suggestion in Hung and Wang (2009). For illustration, first consider a situation where there are two continuous co-primary endpoints. As seen in Fig. 2.5, the overall power is lowest (because the corresponding sample size is highest) when there are equal standardized effect sizes and zero correlation among the endpoints. So that, with a common value of $c^* = c_1^* = c_2^*$ (i.e., $\delta = \delta_1 = \delta_2$) in the overall power function, we could set

$$1 - \beta = \Phi_2(-c^*, -c^* \mid \rho^{12} = 0) = \left\{\Phi(-c^*)\right\}^2 \tag{2.6}$$

where $c^* = z_\alpha - \sqrt{\kappa n}\delta$. Solving (2.6) for n provides the conservative sample size n_{CNSV} given by

$$n_{CNSV} \geq \frac{(z_\alpha + z_\gamma)^2}{\kappa\delta^2}$$

where $\gamma = 1 - (1 - \beta)^{1/2}$.

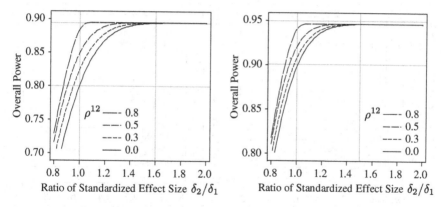

Fig. 2.6 Behavior of overall power $1 - \beta$ as a function of δ_2/δ_1 for a given equal sample size per group $n = n_T = n_C$ (i.e., $r = 1.0$) to detect superiority for endpoint 1 with the targeted individual power $1 - \gamma$ of $0.8^{1/3}$ (the *left panel*) and $0.9^{1/3}$ (the *right panel*) for a one-sided test at the significance level of $\alpha = 0.025$

In practice, one challenge is how to select a common value of c^*. The most conservative way is to choose a smaller value of either c_1^* or c_2^*. This may provide a sample size large enough to detect the joint superiority for both endpoints. Now calculate a sample size n required to detect superiority for endpoint 1, with the targeted individual power $1 - \gamma$ at the significance level of α assuming $\rho^{12} = 0$, i.e., $n_1 = (z_\alpha + z_\gamma)^2/(\kappa\delta_1^2)$, where $\delta_1 \le \delta_2$. The overall power $1 - \beta$ under n_1 is given as

$$1 - \beta = \Phi_2(-c_1^*, -c_2^* \mid \rho^{12} = 0) = \Phi(-c_1^*)\Phi(-c_2^*)$$

where $c_1^* = -z_\gamma$ and $c_2^* = z_\alpha - (\delta_2/\delta_1)(z_\alpha + z_\gamma)$. Therefore, the overall power can be expressed as a function of ratio of the standardized effect sizes.

Figure 2.6 illustrates the behavior of overall power $1 - \beta$ as a function of δ_2/δ_1 for a given equal sample size per group $n = n_T = n_C$ (i.e., $r = 1.0$) to detect superiority for endpoint 1 with the targeted individual power $1 - \gamma$ of $0.8^{1/3}$ and $0.9^{1/3}$ for a one-sided test at the significance level of $\alpha = 0.025$.

For the case of $1 - \gamma = 0.8^{1/2}$, the figure illustrates that the overall power increases toward $0.8^{1/2}$ as the ratio δ_2/δ_1 increases. In particular when the ratio δ_2/δ_1 is roughly greater than 1.6, the overall power almost reaches $0.8^{1/2}$. This is because the individual power for endpoint 2 is very close to one ($\Phi(-c_2^*) \to 1$) under the given sample size calculated for endpoint 1 and the overall power depends greatly on the smaller difference. For the case of $1 - \gamma = 0.9^{1/2}$, when the ratio δ_2/δ_1 is roughly greater than 1.4, then the overall power reaches $0.9^{1/2}$. From this result, if we observe a large difference in the values of δ_1 and δ_2, roughly $\delta_2/\delta_1 > 1.5$, then we could calculate the conservative sample size given by

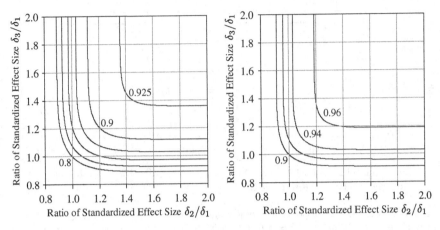

Fig. 2.7 Behavior of overall power $1-\beta$ for three co-primary endpoints as a function of standardized effect sizes for a given equal sample size per group $n = n_T = n_C$ (i.e., $r = 1.0$) to detect superiority for endpoint 1 with the targeted individual power $1 - \gamma$ of $0.8^{1/3}$ (the *left panel*) and $0.9^{1/3}$ (the *right panel*) for a one-sided test at the significance level of $\alpha = 0.025$

$$n'_{CNSV} \geq \max\left(\frac{(z_\alpha + z_\beta)^2}{\kappa\delta_1^2}, \frac{(z_\alpha + z_\beta)^2}{\kappa\delta_2^2}\right).$$

Next we consider a more general situation where there are more than two endpoints. Similarly we calculate a sample size n to detect superiority for endpoint 1, with the targeted individual power $1 - \gamma = (1 - \beta)^{1/K}$ at the significance level of α assuming $\rho^{kk'} = 0$ i.e., $n_1 = (z_\alpha + z_\gamma)^2/(\kappa\delta_1^2)$, where $\delta_1 \leq \cdots \leq \delta_K$. Then the overall power $1 - \beta$ under n_1 is given as

$$1 - \beta = \Phi_K(-c_1^*, \ldots, -c_K^* \mid \rho^{12} = \cdots = \rho^{K-1,K} = 0) = \Phi(-c_1^*) \cdots \Phi(-c_K^*) \tag{2.7}$$

where $c_1^* = -z_\gamma$ and $c_K^* = z_\alpha - (\delta_K/\delta_1)(z_\alpha + z_\gamma)$. Figure 2.7 illustrates the behavior of overall power for three co-primary endpoints as a function of δ_2/δ_1 and δ_3/δ_1 for a given equal sample size per group $n = n_T = n_C$ (i.e., $r = 1.0$) to detect superiority for endpoint 1 with the individual power $1 - \gamma$ of $0.8^{1/3}$ and $0.9^{1/3}$ for a one-sided test at the significance level of $\alpha = 0.025$.

For the case of $1-\gamma = 0.8^{1/3}$, the figure illustrates that the overall power increases toward $0.8^{1/2}$ as the ratio δ_2/δ_1 increases. In particular when both the ratio δ_2/δ_1 and δ_3/δ_1 are roughly greater than 1.5, the overall power almost reaches $0.8^{1/3}$. For the case of $1 - \gamma = 0.9^{1/3}$, when the both ratios are roughly greater than 1.4, the overall power almost reaches $0.9^{1/3}$. From this result, if we observe a large difference in the values of effect sizes, we could calculate the conservative sample size given by

$$n'_{CNSV} \geq \max\left(\frac{(z_\alpha + z_\beta)^2}{\kappa\delta_k^2}\right). \tag{2.8}$$

One question that arises is how large δ_k/δ_1 should be when the conservative sample size (2.8) is considered. To provide a reference value for δ_k/δ_1, the overall power (2.7) is set to be at least $1 - \beta'$, i.e.,

$$(1 - r)\Phi(-z_\alpha + \delta_2/\delta_1(z_\alpha + z_\gamma)) \cdots \Phi(-z_\alpha + \delta_K/\delta_1(z_\alpha + z_\gamma)) > 1 - \beta' \quad (2.9)$$

and then the values of δ_k/δ_1 can be found satisfying the above inequality. For example, we consider a situation of $K = 2$. Solving (2.9) for δ_2/δ_1 gives

$$\frac{\delta_2}{\delta_1} > \frac{\Phi^{-1}\left(\frac{1 - \beta'}{1 - \gamma}\right) + z_\alpha}{z_\gamma + z_\alpha}. \quad (2.10)$$

If the target overall power $1 - \beta = 0.80$ and then the overall power is set to be at least greater than $1 - \beta' = 0.894$ as $1 - \gamma = \sqrt{0.8}$, by substituting these values into above inequality, we have $\delta_2/\delta_1 > 1.639$ with $\alpha = 0.025$. So that, when the one standardized effect size is large enough (or small enough) compared with the other, i.e., $\delta_2/\delta_1 > 1.639$, we may use the sample size equation (2.8). However, if $1 - \beta' = 0.8944$, $\delta_2/\delta_1 > 1.859$. Note that the ratio of standardized effect size will depend on a precision of decimal degree of $1 - \beta'$.

In addition, we discuss a more general situation with K endpoints. For simplicity, we assume $\delta_2 = \cdots = \delta_K$. Solving (2.9) for δ_k/δ_1, we have

$$\frac{\delta_k}{\delta_1} > \frac{\Phi^{-1}\left(\left(\frac{1 - \beta'}{1 - \gamma}\right)^{\frac{1}{K-1}}\right) + z_\alpha}{z_\gamma + z_\alpha}.$$

Table 2.3 Reference values for ratio of standardized effect sizes for conservative sample sizing (2.8) with equal effect sizes $\delta_2 = \cdots = \delta_K$. $1 - \beta'$ is calculated by truncating the numbers beyond the fourth decimal point

Number of endpoints	Targeted overall $1 - \beta$			
	0.80	$(1 - \beta')$	0.90	$(1 - \beta')$
2	1.639	(0.894)	1.432	(0.948)
3	1.564	(0.928)	1.388	(0.965)
4	1.436	(0.945)	1.648	(0.974)
5	1.453	(0.956)	1.394	(0.979)
6	1.397	(0.963)	1.276	(0.982)
7	1.355	(0.968)	1.403	(0.985)
8	1.352	(0.972)	1.212	(0.986)
9	1.333	(0.975)	1.262	(0.988)
10	1.274	(0.977)	1.226	(0.989)

For example, consider a situation of $K = 3$. If the target overall power $1 - \beta = 0.80$ and the overall power is set to be at least greater than $1 - \beta' = 0.928$ as $1 - \gamma = 0.8^{1/3}$, we have $\delta_k/\delta_1 > 1.564$ with $\alpha = 0.025$. So that we may use the sample size equation (2.8) when both of the ratio of standardized effect sizes are larger than 1.564.

Table 2.3 shows typical reference values for ratio of standardized effect sizes given by (2.9) with equal effect sizes $\delta_2 = \cdots = \delta_K$ when the conservative sample size (2.8) is considered.

2.6 Example

We illustrate the sample size calculations based on a clinical trial evaluating interventions for Alzheimer's disease. In Alzheimer's clinical trials, the change from the baseline in the ADAS-cog (the Alzheimer's Disease Assessment Scale-cognitive subscale) score and the CIBIC-plus (Clinician's Interview-Based Impression of Change, plus caregiver) at the last observed time point are commonly used as co-primary endpoints (e.g., Peskind et al. 2006; Rogers et al. 1998; Rösler et al. 1999; Tariot et al. 2000). In a 24-week, double-blind, placebo controlled trial of donepezil in patients with Alzheimer's disease in Rogers et al. (1998), the absolute values of the standardized effect size (with 95 % confidence interval) were estimated as 0.47 (0.24, 0.69) for ADAS-cog (δ_1) and 0.48 (0.25 0.70) for CIBIC-plus (δ_2). We use these estimates to define an alternative hypothesis to size a future trial. The sample sizes were calculated using the method based on the known variance to detect the standardized effect sizes $0.20 < \delta_1$, $\delta_2 < 0.70$ to achieve the overall power of $1 - \beta = 0.80$ at $\alpha = 0.025$, with $\rho^{12} = 0, 0.3, 0.5$, and 0.8 as the correlation between the two endpoints.

Figure 2.8 displays the contour plots of the sample sizes per group with two effect sizes δ_1 and δ_2 and correlation ρ^{12}. The figure displays how the sample size behaves as the two effect sizes and the correlations vary; when the effect sizes are approximately equal, the required sample size varies with the correlation. When one effect size is relativity smaller (or larger) than the other, the sample size is nearly determined by the smaller effect size, and does not depend greatly on the correlation. The correlation ρ^{12} is assumed to range between $-1 < \rho^{12} < 0.35$ by Offen et al. (2007) and $\rho^{12} = 0.5$ (as a trial value) by Xiong et al. 2005. As the baseline case of $(\delta_1, \delta_2) = (0.47, 0.48)$, the sample sizes per group for $\rho^{12} = 0, 0.3, 0.5$, and 0.8 were 92, 90, 87, and 82, respectively.

2.7 Summary

This chapter provides an overview of the concepts and technical fundamentals regarding power and sample size calculation for clinical trials with co-primary continuous endpoints when the alternative hypothesis is joint effects on all endpoints. The chapter also introduces conservative sample sizing strategies. Our major findings are as follows:

- There is an advantage of incorporating the correlation among endpoints into the power and sample size calculations with co-primary continuous endpoints. In general without design adjustments, the power is lower with additional endpoints, but can be improved by incorporating the correlation into the calculation (assuming a positive correlation). Thus incorporating the correlation into the sample size calculation may lead to a reduction in sample sizes. The reduction in sample size is greater with a greater number of endpoints, especially when the standardized effect sizes are approximately equal among the endpoints. For example, when the endpoints are positively correlated (correlation up to 0.8), with the power of 0.8

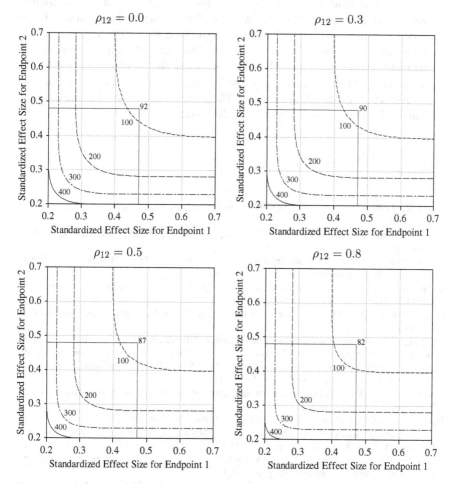

Fig. 2.8 Contour plot of the sample size (per group) for standardized effect sizes of endpoint 1 (SIB-J) and endpoint 2 (CIBIC plus-J) with $\rho^{12} = 0.0, 0.3, 0.5,$ and 0.8. The sample size was calculated to detect the superiority for all the endpoints with the overall power of $1 - \beta = 0.80$ for a one-sided test at the significance level of $\alpha = 0.025$

at the significant level of 0.025, there is approximately 11 % reduction in the case of two co-primary endpoints and 16 % reduction in the case of three co-primary endpoints, compared to the sample size calculated under the assumption of zero correlations among the endpoints.

- In most situations, the required sample size per group for co-primary continuous endpoints calculated using the method based on the assumption that variance is unknown is one participant larger than the method based on the assumption that the variance is known. This is very similar to results seen for a single continuous endpoint.
- When the standardized effect sizes for the endpoints are unequal, then the advantage of incorporating the correlation into sample size is less dramatic as the required sample size is primarily determined by the smaller standardized effect size and does not greatly depend on the correlation. In this situation, the sample size equation for co-primary continuous endpoints can be simplified using the equation for a single continuous endpoint, as given by Eq. (2.8). When the standardized effect sizes among endpoints are approximately equal, then the sample size method assuming zero correlation described in Hung and Wang (2009) may be used as the power is minimized with the equal standardized effect sizes.

References

Berger RL (1982) Multiparameter hypothesis testing and acceptance sampling. Technometrics 24:295–300

Bretz F, Hothorn T, Westfall P (2011) Multiple comparisons using R. Chapman & Hall/CRC, Boca Raton

Chuang-Stein C, Stryszak P, Dmitrienko A, Offen W (2007) Challenge of multiple co-primary endpoints: a new approach. Stat Med 26:1181–1192

Eaton ML, Muirhead RJ (2007) On a multiple endpoints testing problem. J Stat Plann Infer 137:3416–3429

Hung HM, Wang SJ (2009) Some controversial multiple testing problems in regulatory applications. J Biopharm Stat 19:1–11

International conference on harmonisation of technical requirements for registration of pharmaceuticals for human use. ICH tripartite guideline. Statistical principles for clinical trials. 1998. http://www.ich.org/fileadmin/Public_Web_Site/ICH_Products/Guidelines/Efficacy/E9/Step4/E9_Guideline.pdf Accessed 9 June 2014

Johnson NL, Kotz S (1972) Distributions in statistics: continuous multivariate distributions. Wiley, New York

Julious SA (2009) Sample sizes for clinical trials. Chapman & Hall, Boca Raton

Offen W, Chuang-Stein C, Dmitrienko A, Littman G, Maca J, Meyerson L, Muirhead R, Stryszak P, Boddy A, Chen K, Copley-Merriman K, Dere W, Givens S, Hall D, Henry D, Jackson JD, Krishen A, Liu T, Ryder S, Sankoh AJ, Wang J, Yeh CH (2007) Multiple co-primary endpoints: medical and statistical solutions. Drug Inf J 41:31–46

Peskind ER, Potkin SG, Pomara N, Ott BR, Graham SM, Olin JT, McDonald S (2006) Memantine treatment in mild to moderate Alzheimer disease: a 24-week randomized, controlled trial. Am J Geriatr Psychiatry 14:704–715

Rogers SL, Farlow MR, Doody RS, Mohs R, Friedhoff LT (1998) The Donepezil Study Group. A 24-week, double-blind, placebo-controlled trial of donepezil in patients with Alzheimer's disease. Neurology 50:136–145

Rösler M, Anand R, Cicin-Sain A, Gauthier S, Agid Y, Dal-Bianco P, Stähelin HB, Hartman R, Gharabawi M (1999) Efficacy and safety of rivastigmine in patients with Alzheimer's disease: international randomised controlled trial. Br Med J 318:633–640

Senn S, Bretz F (2007) Power and sample size when multiple endpoints are considered

Sozu T, Kanou T, Hamada C, Yoshimura I (2006) Power and sample size calculations in clinical trials with multiple primary variables. Japan J Biometrics 27:83–96

Sozu T, Sugimoto T, Hamasaki T (2011) Sample size determination in superiority clinical trials with multiple co-primary correlated endpoints. J Biopharm Stat 21:650–668

Tariot PN, Solomon PR, Morris JC, Kershaw P, Lilienfeld S, Ding C (2000) The Galantamine USA Study Group. A 5-month, randomized, placebo-controlled trial of galantamine in AD. Neurology 54:2269–2276

Westfall PH, Tobias RD, Wolfinger RD (2011) Multiple comparisons and multiple tests using SAS, 2nd edn. SAS Institute Inc, Cary

Xiong C, Yu K, Gao F, Yan Y, Zhang Z (2005) Power and sample size for clinical trials when efficacy is required in multiple endpoints: application to an Alzheimer's treatment trial. Clin Trials 2:387–393

Chapter 3
Binary Co-primary Endpoints

Abstract In this chapter, we provide methods for power and sample size calculation for clinical trials with multiple co-primary binary endpoints. On the basis of three association measures among the multiple binary endpoints, we discuss five methods for power and sample size calculation: the asymptotic normal method with and without a continuity correction, the arcsine method with and without a continuity correction, and the Fisher's exact method. We evaluate the behavior of the sample size and empirical power associated with the methods. We also provide numerical examples to illustrate the methods.

Keywords Arcsine transformation · Association measures · Continuity correction · Fisher's exact test · Multivariate Bernoulli

3.1 Introduction

Consider a randomized clinical trial comparing two interventions with n_T subjects in the test group and n_C subjects in the control group. There are $K (\geq 2)$ co-primary binary (or dichotomized) endpoints. Let the responses for n_T subjects in the test group be denoted by Y_{Tjk}, $j = 1, \ldots, n_T$ and those for n_C subjects in the control group, by Y_{Cjk}, $j = 1, \ldots, n_C$.

We are interested in estimating the differences in the proportions $\pi_{Tk} - \pi_{Ck}$. A positive value of $\pi_{Tk} - \pi_{Ck}$ indicates an intervention benefit. We assert the superiority of the test intervention over the control in terms of all K primary endpoints if and only if $\mu_{Tk} - \mu_{Ck} > 0$ for all $k = 1, \ldots, K$. Thus, the hypotheses for testing are

$$H_0 : \pi_{Tk} - \pi_{Ck} \leq 0 \text{ for at least one } k,$$
$$H_1 : \pi_{Tk} - \pi_{Ck} > 0 \text{ for all } k.$$

In testing the preceding hypotheses, the null hypothesis H_0 is rejected if and only if all of the null hypotheses associated with each of the K primary endpoints are rejected at a significance level of α. Although, in many clinical trials, the most commonly used measure is a difference in the proportions between two interventions as described above, risk ratio and odds ratio are also frequently used in clinical trials to measure a

© The Author(s) 2015
T. Sozu et al., *Sample Size Determination in Clinical Trials with Multiple Endpoints*,
SpringerBriefs in Statistics, DOI 10.1007/978-3-319-22005-5_3

risk reduction. The power and sample size calculation for these measures are given in Appendixs A1 and A2 respectively.

In general, there are three association measures between a pair of binary endpoints: (i) the correlation of a multivariate Bernoulli distribution, (ii) the odds ratio, and (iii) the correlation of a latent multivariate normal distribution. Please see, e.g., Johnson et al. (1997) for the definition of the multivariate Bernoulli distribution. The choice of an association measure may depend on several factors including the nature and characteristics of endpoints and the statistical methods used for data analysis.

(i) Correlation of a Multivariate Bernoulli Distribution

Suppose that the vectors of responses $Y_{Tj} = (Y_{Tj1}, \ldots, Y_{TjK})^T$ and $Y_{Cj} = (Y_{Cj1}, \ldots, Y_{CjK})^T$ are independently distributed as K-variate Bernoulli distributions with $E[Y_{Tjk}] = \pi_{Tk}$, $E[Y_{Cjk}] = \pi_{Ck}$, $var[Y_{Tjk}] = \pi_{Tk}\theta_{Tk}$, and $var[Y_{Cjk}] = \pi_{Ck}\theta_{Ck}$, where $\theta_{Tk} = 1 - \pi_{Tk}$ and $\theta_{Ck} = 1 - \pi_{Ck}$. The association measures between the kth and k'th endpoints for Y_{Tjk} and Y_{Cjk}, $\mathrm{corr}[Y_{Tjk}, Y_{Tjk'}]$ and $\mathrm{corr}[Y_{Cjk}, Y_{Cjk'}]$, are given as a correlation of a multivariate Bernoulli distribution, which are

$$\tau_T^{kk'} = \frac{\phi_T^{kk'} - \pi_{Tk}\pi_{Tk'}}{\sqrt{\pi_{Tk}\theta_{Tk}\pi_{Tk'}\theta_{Tk'}}} \quad \text{and} \quad \tau_C^{kk'} = \frac{\phi_C^{kk'} - \pi_{Ck}\pi_{Ck'}}{\sqrt{\pi_{Ck}\theta_{Ck}\pi_{Ck'}\theta_{Ck'}}}$$

for all $k \neq k'$ ($1 \leq k < k' \leq K$), respectively, where $\phi_T^{kk'}$ and $\phi_C^{kk'}$ are the joint probabilities of the kth and k'th endpoints for Y_{Tjk} and Y_{Cjk}, given by $\phi_T^{kk'} = \mathrm{Pr}[Y_{Tjk} = 1, Y_{Tjk'} = 1]$ and $\phi_C^{kk'} = \mathrm{Pr}[Y_{Cjk} = 1, Y_{Cjk'} = 1]$ respectively. Note that since $0 < \pi_{Tk}, \pi_{Tk'} < 1$ and $0 < \pi_{Ck}, \pi_{Ck'} < 1$, $\tau_T^{kk'}$ and $\tau_C^{kk'}$ are bounded below by

$$\max\left(-\sqrt{\frac{\pi_{Tk}\pi_{Tk'}}{\theta_{Tk}\theta_{Tk'}}}, -\sqrt{\frac{\theta_{Tk}\theta_{Tk'}}{\pi_{Tk}\pi_{Tk'}}}\right) \quad \text{and} \quad \max\left(-\sqrt{\frac{\pi_{Ck}\pi_{Ck'}}{\theta_{Ck}\theta_{Ck'}}}, -\sqrt{\frac{\theta_{Ck}\theta_{Ck'}}{\pi_{Ck}\pi_{Ck'}}}\right)$$

and above by

$$\min\left(\sqrt{\frac{\pi_{Tk}\theta_{Tk'}}{\pi_{Tk'}\theta_{Tk}}}, \sqrt{\frac{\pi_{Tk'}\theta_{Tk}}{\pi_{Tk}\theta_{Tk'}}}\right) \quad \text{and} \quad \min\left(\sqrt{\frac{\pi_{Ck}\theta_{Ck'}}{\pi_{Ck'}\theta_{Ck}}}, \sqrt{\frac{\pi_{Ck'}\theta_{Ck}}{\pi_{Ck}\theta_{Ck'}}}\right)$$

(Emrich and Piedmonte 1991; Prentice 1988).

(ii) Odds Ratio

The association measures between the kth and k'th endpoints for Y_{Tjk} and Y_{Cjk} are given as odds ratios, which are

$$\psi_T^{kk'} = \frac{\phi_T^{kk'}(1 - \pi_{Tk} - \pi_{Tk'} + \phi_T^{kk'})}{(\pi_{Tk} - \phi_T^{kk'})(\pi_{Tk'} - \phi_T^{kk'})} \quad \text{and} \quad \psi_C^{kk'} = \frac{\phi_C^{kk'}(1 - \pi_{Ck} - \pi_{Ck'} + \phi_C^{kk'})}{(\pi_{Ck} - \phi_C^{kk'})(\pi_{Ck'} - \phi_C^{kk'})}$$

respectively.

(iii) Correlation of a Latent Multivariate Normal Distribution

Suppose that the vectors of responses Y_{Tj} and Y_{Cj} are dichotomized random variables of continuous unobserved latent variables $X_{Tj} = (X_{Tj1}, \ldots, X_{TjK})^T$ and $X_{Cj} = (X_{Cj1}, \ldots, X_{CjK})^T$, respectively. X_{Tj} and X_{Cj} are distributed as K-variate normal distributions with correlations $\rho_T^{kk'}$ and $\rho_C^{kk'}$, respectively. The joint probabilities $\phi_T^{kk'}$ and $\phi_C^{kk'}$ are given by

$$\phi_T^{kk'} = \int_{-\infty}^{\infty} \cdots \int_{g_{Tk}}^{\infty} \cdots \int_{g_{Tk'}}^{\infty} \cdots \int_{-\infty}^{\infty} f(x_T; \rho_T^{kk'}) dx_{T1} \ldots dx_{TK}$$

and

$$\phi_C^{kk'} = \int_{-\infty}^{\infty} \cdots \int_{g_{Ck}}^{\infty} \cdots \int_{g_{Ck'}}^{\infty} \cdots \int_{-\infty}^{\infty} f(x_C; \rho_C^{kk'}) dx_{C1} \ldots dx_{CK}$$

respectively, where functions $f(x_T; \rho_T^{kk'})$ and $f(x_C; \rho_C^{kk'})$ are the joint density functions of X_{Tj} and X_{Cj}, respectively, with $\pi_{Tk} = \Pr[X_{Tjk} \geq g_{Tk}] = \Pr[Y_{Tjk} = 1]$, $\pi_{Ck} = \Pr[X_{Cjk} \geq g_{Ck}] = \Pr[Y_{Cjk} = 1]$, and

$$Y_{Tjk} = \begin{cases} 1, & X_{Tjk} \geq g_{Tk}, \\ 0, & X_{Tjk} < g_{Tk}, \end{cases} \quad \text{and} \quad Y_{Cjk} = \begin{cases} 1, & X_{Cjk} \geq g_{Ck}, \\ 0, & X_{Cjk} < g_{Ck}. \end{cases}$$

3.2 Test Statistics and Power

3.2.1 Chi-Square Test and Related Test Statistics

We consider four testing methods using an asymptotic normal approximation with and without a continuity correction (CC). The test statistic for each primary endpoint is given as follows:

(1) One-sided chi-square test without CC (Pearson 1900)

$$Z_k = \frac{p_{Tk} - p_{Ck}}{\sqrt{\left(\dfrac{1}{n_T} + \dfrac{1}{n_C}\right) p_k(1 - p_k)}}, \tag{3.1}$$

where p_{Tk} and p_{Ck} are the sample proportions given by

$$p_{Tk} = \frac{1}{n_T} \sum_{j=1}^{n_T} Y_{Tjk} \quad \text{and} \quad p_{Ck} = \frac{1}{n_C} \sum_{j=1}^{n_C} Y_{Cjk}; \quad p_k = \frac{n_T p_{Tk} + n_C p_{Ck}}{n_T + n_C}.$$

(2) One-sided chi-square test with CC (Yates 1934)

$$Z_k = \frac{p_{Tk} - p_{Ck} - \dfrac{1}{2}\left(\dfrac{1}{n_T} + \dfrac{1}{n_C}\right)}{\sqrt{\left(\dfrac{1}{n_T} + \dfrac{1}{n_C}\right) p_k(1 - p_k)}}. \tag{3.2}$$

(3) Arcsine root transformation method without CC (Bartlett 1947)

$$Z_k = \frac{\sin^{-1}\sqrt{p_{Tk}} - \sin^{-1}\sqrt{p_{Ck}}}{\dfrac{1}{2}\sqrt{\dfrac{1}{n_T} + \dfrac{1}{n_C}}}. \tag{3.3}$$

(4) Arcsine root transformation method with CC (Walters 1979)

$$Z_k = \frac{\sin^{-1}\sqrt{p_{Tk} - \dfrac{1}{2n_T}} - \sin^{-1}\sqrt{p_{Ck} + \dfrac{1}{2n_C}}}{\dfrac{1}{2}\sqrt{\dfrac{1}{n_T} + \dfrac{1}{n_C}}}. \tag{3.4}$$

If $p_{Tk} - 1/2n_T < 0$ (i.e., $Y_{Tjk} = 0$), this term is replaced by 0. Similarly, if $p_{Ck} + 1/2n_C > 1$ (i.e., $Y_{Cjk} = n_C$), this term is replaced by 1. These replacements should be carefully considered when calculating the test statistics (3.4) during data analysis.

As an illustration, the overall power function for statistic (3.1) can be written as

$$1 - \beta = \Pr\left[\bigcap_{k=1}^{K}\{Z_k > z_\alpha\} \,\middle|\, H_1\right] = \Pr\left[\bigcap_{k=1}^{K}\{Z_k^* > c_k^*\} \,\middle|\, H_1\right] \tag{3.5}$$

where

$$Z_k^* = \frac{p_{Tk} - p_{Ck} - \delta_k}{\sqrt{\dfrac{\kappa\pi_{Tk}\theta_{Tk} + (1 - \kappa)\pi_{Ck}\theta_{Ck}}{\kappa n}}}$$

$$c_k^* = \frac{1}{\sqrt{(\kappa/(1 - \kappa))\pi_{Tk}\theta_{Tk} + \pi_{Ck}\theta_{Ck}}}\left(\sqrt{\frac{((1 - \kappa)\pi_{Tk} + \kappa\pi_{Ck})((1 - \kappa)\theta_{Tk} + \kappa\theta_{Ck})}{1 - \kappa}}z_\alpha - \sqrt{\kappa n}\delta_k\right), \tag{3.6}$$

$\delta_k = \pi_{Tk} - \pi_{Ck}$, $r = n_C/n_T$, $n = n_T$, $\kappa = r/(1 + r)$, and p_k is replaced by $\bar{p}_k = (1 - \kappa)\pi_{Tk} + \kappa\pi_{Ck}$.

Since $E[Z_k^*] = 0$ and $\mathrm{var}[Z_k^*] = 1$, the vector of $(Z_1^*, \ldots, Z_K^*)^T$ is approximately distributed as a K-variate normal distribution, $N_K(\mathbf{0}, \rho_{Z^*})$, where the off-diagonal element of ρ_{Z^*} is given by

$$\rho_D^{kk'} = \frac{\kappa\,\mathrm{corr}[Y_{Tjk}, Y_{Tjk'}]\sqrt{\pi_{Tk}\theta_{Tk}\pi_{Tk'}\theta_{Tk'}} + (1 - \kappa)\,\mathrm{corr}[Y_{Cjk}, Y_{Cjk'}]\sqrt{\pi_{Ck}\theta_{Ck}\pi_{Ck'}\theta_{Ck'}}}{\sqrt{\kappa\pi_{Tk}\theta_{Tk} + (1 - \kappa)\pi_{Ck}\theta_{Ck}}\sqrt{\kappa\pi_{Tk'}\theta_{Tk'} + (1 - \kappa)\pi_{Ck'}\theta_{Ck'}}}.$$

The definitions of $\mathrm{corr}[Y_{Tjk}, Y_{Tjk'}]$ and $\mathrm{corr}[Y_{Cjk}, Y_{Cjk'}]$ depend on the assumed model for the response variables Y_{Tj} and Y_{Cj}. For example, when the K-variate Bernoulli distribution is assumed,

$$\rho_D^{kk'} = \frac{\kappa(\phi_T^{kk'} - \pi_{Tk}\pi_{Tk'}) + (1-\kappa)(\phi_C^{kk'} - \pi_{Ck}\pi_{Ck'})}{\sqrt{\kappa\pi_{Tk}\theta_{Tk} + (1-\kappa)\pi_{Ck}\theta_{Ck}}\sqrt{\kappa\pi_{Tk'}\theta_{Tk'} + (1-\kappa)\pi_{Ck'}\theta_{Ck'}}}.$$

The overall power function of (3.5) is calculated using $\Phi_K(-c_1^*, \ldots, -c_K^*)$, where Φ_K is the cumulative distribution function of $N_K(\mathbf{0}, \rho_{Z*})$. The corresponding c_k^* and $\rho_D^{kk'}$ for the overall power functions for other testing methods are summarized in Table 3.1 (Sozu et al. 2010, 2011). We refer to the sample size calculations using these test statistics as (1) the chi-square method (without CC), (2) the chi-square method with CC, (3) the arcsine method (without CC), and (4) the arcsine method with CC, respectively.

The normal approximation discussed here may work well in larger sample sizes, but not when events are rare or when sample sizes are small. In such situations, one alternative is to consider more direct ways of calculating the sample size without using a normal approximation, which will be discussed in Sect. 3.2.2. However, such direct methods are computationally difficult, particularly for the large sample sizes and thus can be impractical to utilize. The utility of using the normal approximation is compared with the direct methods in Appendix B.

3.2.2 Fisher's Exact Test

Fisher's exact test is widely used to evaluate the difference in two proportions, particularly when events are rare or very common resulting in small numbers in cells of a 2×2 table. We outline the overall power calculations for Fisher's exact test.

Under the null hypothesis, when the sum of the observed number of $\sum_{j=1}^{n_T} Y_{Tjk} + \sum_{j=1}^{n_C} Y_{Cjk} = Y_k$ is fixed, $\sum_{j=1}^{n_T} Y_{Tjk} = Y_{Tk}$ is conditionally distributed as a hypergeometric distribution. The one-sided p-value corresponding to the kth primary endpoint is given by

$$P_k = \sum_{Y_{Tk}}^{\min(n_T, Y_k)} \binom{Y_k}{Y_{Tk}} \binom{n_T + n_C - Y_k}{n_T - Y_{Tk}} \Big/ \binom{n_T + n_C}{n_T}.$$

The conditional power is given by $\Pr\left[\bigcap_{k=1}^{K}\{P_k < \alpha\} \mid H_1\right]$. The expected overall power can be calculated using Monte Carlo integration. The sample size required to achieve the desired overall power is the smallest integer where the subsequent sample sizes have more power than $1 - \beta$, considering the discrete nature of the binomial distribution. Hereinafter, the sample size calculation for Fisher's exact test is referred to as the exact method.

Table 3.1 c_k^* in the overall power function of $\Phi_K(-c_1^*, \ldots, -c_K^*)$ and $\rho_D^{kk'}$, the off-diagonal element of ρ_{Z^*}, in $N_K(\mathbf{0}, \rho_{Z^*})$

Method	c_k^*	$\rho_D^{kk'}$
Chi-square method	$\dfrac{v_{k0}z_\alpha - \sqrt{\kappa n}\,\delta_k}{v_k}$	$\dfrac{\kappa\,\mathrm{corr}[Y_{Tjk}, Y_{Tjk'}]\sqrt{\pi_{Tk}\theta_{Tk}\pi_{Tk'}\theta_{Tk'}} + (1-\kappa)\mathrm{corr}[Y_{Cjk}, Y_{Cjk'}]\sqrt{\pi_{Ck}\theta_{Ck}\pi_{Ck'}\theta_{Ck'}}}{\sqrt{\kappa\pi_{Tk}\theta_{Tk} + (1-\kappa)\pi_{Ck}\theta_{Ck}}\,\sqrt{\kappa\pi_{Tk'}\theta_{Tk'} + (1-\kappa)\pi_{Ck'}\theta_{Ck'}}}$
Chi-square method with CC	$\dfrac{v_{k0}z_\alpha - \sqrt{\kappa n}\,\delta_k}{v_k} + \dfrac{1}{2v_k\sqrt{\kappa n}}$	
Arcsine method	$z_\alpha - 2\sqrt{\kappa n}\left(\sin^{-1}\sqrt{\pi_{Tk}} - \sin^{-1}\sqrt{\pi_{Ck}}\right)$	$\kappa\,\mathrm{corr}[Y_{Tjk}, Y_{Tjk'}] + (1-\kappa)\mathrm{corr}[Y_{Cjk}, Y_{Cjk'}]$
Arcsine method with CC	$z_\alpha - \sqrt{\kappa n}\dfrac{\left(\sin^{-1}\sqrt{\pi_{Tk}^c} - \sin^{-1}\sqrt{\pi_{Ck}^c}\right)}{\sqrt{\dfrac{\kappa\pi_{Tk}\theta_{Tk}}{\pi_{Tk}^c\theta_{Tk}^c} + \dfrac{(1-\kappa)\pi_{Ck}\theta_{Ck}}{\pi_{Ck}^c\theta_{Ck}^c}}}$	$\dfrac{\kappa\,\mathrm{corr}[Y_{Tjk}, Y_{Tjk'}]\sqrt{\dfrac{\pi_{Tk}\theta_{Tk}\pi_{Tk'}\theta_{Tk'}}{\pi_{Tk}^c\theta_{Tk}^c\pi_{Tk'}^c\theta_{Tk'}^c}} + (1-\kappa)\mathrm{corr}[Y_{Cjk}, Y_{Cjk'}]\sqrt{\dfrac{\pi_{Ck}\theta_{Ck}\pi_{Ck'}\theta_{Ck'}}{\pi_{Ck}^c\theta_{Ck}^c\pi_{Ck'}^c\theta_{Ck'}^c}}}{\sqrt{\dfrac{\kappa\pi_{Tk}\theta_{Tk}}{\pi_{Tk}^c\theta_{Tk}^c} + \dfrac{(1-\kappa)\pi_{Ck}\theta_{Ck}}{\pi_{Ck}^c\theta_{Ck}^c}}\,\sqrt{\dfrac{\kappa\pi_{Tk'}\theta_{Tk'}}{\pi_{Tk'}^c\theta_{Tk'}^c} + \dfrac{(1-\kappa)\pi_{Ck'}\theta_{Ck'}}{\pi_{Ck'}^c\theta_{Ck'}^c}}}$

$v_{k0} = \sqrt{((1-\kappa)\pi_{Tk} + \kappa\pi_{Ck})((1-\kappa)\theta_{Tk} + \kappa\theta_{Ck})}, \quad v_k = \sqrt{\kappa\pi_{Tk}\theta_{Tk} + (1-\kappa)\pi_{Ck}\theta_{Ck}},$

$\pi_{Tk}^c = \pi_{Tk} - \dfrac{1}{2n}, \quad \theta_{Tk}^c = \theta_{Tk} + \dfrac{1}{2n}, \quad \pi_{Ck}^c = \pi_{Ck} + \dfrac{1}{2n}\left(\dfrac{1-\kappa}{\kappa}\right), \quad \theta_{Ck}^c = \theta_{Ck} - \dfrac{1}{2n}\left(\dfrac{1-\kappa}{\kappa}\right)$

When the exact method is used, extensive computation must be carried out to calculate the overall power and to determine the sample size required to achieve the desired overall power. To reduce the computational burden, the arcsine method with CC may be used, as in the case of a single binary endpoint (Sozu et al. 2010). The overall power function for the arcsine method with CC is given in Table 3.1.

In the sample size calculation, the proportions π_{Tk}, π_{Ck}, and the associations among endpoints must be specified in advance. The choice of an association measure may depend on several factors including the nature and characteristics of endpoints and the statistical methods used for data analysis. All of the three association measures

Table 3.2 Sample size per group ($n = n_T = n_C, r = 1.0$) for two endpoints ($K = 2$) with the overall power of $1 - \beta = 0.80$

Proportions		Method	Correlation τ^{12}				
π_{Tk}	π_{Ck}		0.0	0.3	0.5	0.8	1.0
0.55	0.50	Chi-square	2055 (2094)	2003 (2043)	1951 (1991)	1826 (1866)	1565 (1605)
		Arcsine	2055 (2095)	2003 (2043)	1951 (1991)	1826 (1866)	1565 (1605)
		Exact	2097	2041	1984	1859	1606
0.60	0.50	Chi-square	509 (528)	496 (516)	483 (503)	452 (472)	388 (408)
		Arcsine	509 (529)	496 (516)	483 (503)	452 (472)	388 (407)
		Exact	526	518	498	467	404
0.65	0.50	Chi-square	222 (236)	217 (230)	211 (224)	198 (211)	170 (184)
		Arcsine	223 (236)	217 (230)	211 (224)	198 (211)	170 (183)
		Exact	237	228	224	208	183
0.70	0.50	Chi-square	122 (132)	119 (129)	116 (126)	109 (119)	93 (103)
		Arcsine	122 (132)	119 (129)	116 (126)	109 (118)	93 (103)
		Exact	131	129	127	117	102
0.75	0.50	Chi-square	76 (84)	74 (82)	72 (80)	68 (75)	58 (66)
		Arcsine	76 (83)	74 (82)	72 (80)	67 (75)	58 (66)
		Exact	84	81	78	75	64
0.80	0.50	Chi-square	51 (57)	49 (56)	48 (55)	45 (52)	39 (46)
		Arcsine	50 (57)	49 (55)	48 (54)	45 (51)	38 (45)
		Exact	56	55	54	51	44
0.85	0.50	Chi-square	35 (41)	35 (40)	34 (39)	32 (37)	27 (33)
		Arcsine	35 (40)	34 (39)	33 (39)	31 (36)	27 (32)
		Exact	40	39	38	36	32
0.90	0.50	Chi-square	25 (30)	25 (30)	24 (29)	24 (28)	20 (25)
		Arcsine	24 (29)	24 (29)	23 (28)	22 (27)	19 (24)
		Exact	29	28	28	27	23
0.95	0.50	Chi-square	19 (23)	18 (23)	18 (22)	17 (21)	15 (20)
		Arcsine	17 (21)	17 (21)	16 (20)	15 (19)	13 (17)
		Exact	21	20	20	19	17

The values in parentheses are the sample size per group by the corresponding method with CC in Sect. 3.1 can be estimated from the proportions and joint probabilities of the endpoints. As in the case of the continuous co-primary endpoints, an iterative procedure is required to find the required sample size. Chapter 4 provides a more efficient and practical algorithm for calculating the sample sizes and presents a useful sample size formula with numerical tables.

3.3 Behavior of the Sample Size

We illustrate the behavior of sample sizes calculated by the five methods discussed in the previous sections when there are two ($K = 2$) and three ($K = 3$) co-primary endpoints. The equal sample sizes per group $n = n_T = n_C$ (i.e., $r = 1.0$) were calculated with the overall power of $1 - \beta = 0.80$ when each of the K endpoints is

Table 3.3 Sample size per group ($n = n_T = n_C, r = 1.0$) for two endpoints ($K = 2$) with the overall power of $1 - \beta = 0.80$

Proportions		Method	Correlation τ^{12}				
π_{Tk}	π_{Ck}		0.0	0.3	0.5	0.8	1.0
0.65	0.60	Chi-square	1931 (1971)	1882 (1922)	1834 (1873)	1716 (1756)	1471 (1511)
		Arcsine	1931 (1971)	1882 (1922)	1834 (1873)	1716 (1756)	1471 (1510)
		Exact	1969	1918	1879	1758	1514
0.70	0.60	Chi-square	467 (487)	456 (476)	444 (464)	416 (435)	356 (376)
		Arcsine	467 (487)	455 (475)	444 (463)	415 (435)	356 (376)
		Exact	488	474	463	434	375
0.75	0.60	Chi-square	199 (213)	194 (208)	190 (203)	177 (191)	152 (166)
		Arcsine	199 (212)	194 (207)	189 (202)	177 (190)	152 (165)
		Exact	212	206	202	189	164
0.80	0.60	Chi-square	107 (116)	104 (114)	101 (111)	95 (105)	82 (92)
		Arcsine	106 (116)	103 (113)	101 (110)	94 (104)	81 (91)
		Exact	116	112	110	103	90
0.85	0.60	Chi-square	64 (72)	63 (70)	61 (69)	57 (65)	49 (57)
		Arcsine	63 (71)	61 (69)	60 (68)	56 (64)	48 (56)
		Exact	71	69	67	63	56
0.90	0.60	Chi-square	41 (48)	40 (47)	39 (46)	37 (43)	32 (39)
		Arcsine	40 (46)	39 (45)	38 (44)	35 (42)	30 (37)
		Exact	46	45	44	41	36
0.95	0.60	Chi-square	28 (33)	27 (33)	26 (32)	25 (30)	22 (28)
		Arcsine	25 (30)	24 (30)	24 (29)	22 (28)	19 (25)
		Exact	31	30	29	28	24

The values in parentheses are the sample size per group by the corresponding method with CC

Table 3.4 Sample size per group ($n = n_T = n_C, r = 1.0$) for two endpoints ($K = 2$) with the overall power of $1 - \beta = 0.80$

Proportions		Method	Correlation τ^{12}				
π_{Tk}	π_{Ck}		0.0	0.3	0.5	0.8	1.0
0.75	0.70	Chi-square	1642 (1682)	1601 (1641)	1560 (1599)	1460 (1499)	1251 (1291)
		Arcsine	1641 (1681)	1600 (1640)	1559 (1598)	1458 (1498)	1250 (1290)
		Exact	1680	1640	1599	1498	1292
0.80	0.70	Chi-square	385 (405)	375 (395)	366 (385)	342 (362)	294 (314)
		Arcsine	384 (403)	374 (394)	364 (384)	341 (361)	292 (312)
		Exact	403	393	383	361	311
0.85	0.70	Chi-square	158 (171)	154 (167)	150 (163)	141 (154)	121 (135)
		Arcsine	156 (169)	152 (165)	148 (161)	139 (152)	119 (132)
		Exact	169	165	161	152	131
0.90	0.70	Chi-square	81 (91)	79 (89)	77 (87)	72 (82)	62 (72)
		Arcsine	78 (88)	76 (86)	74 (84)	69 (79)	60 (69)
		Exact	88	86	84	79	69
0.95	0.70	Chi-square	46 (54)	45 (53)	44 (52)	41 (49)	36 (44)
		Arcsine	42 (49)	41 (48)	40 (47)	37 (45)	32 (40)
		Exact	50	49	48	45	39
0.85	0.80	Chi-square	1189 (1229)	1159 (1199)	1129 (1169)	1057 (1096)	906 (946)
		Arcsine	1185 (1225)	1156 (1195)	1126 (1165)	1053 (1093)	903 (942)
		Exact	1224	1194	1165	1093	942
0.90	0.80	Chi-square	261 (281)	255 (274)	248 (268)	232 (252)	199 (219)
		Arcsine	256 (276)	250 (270)	244 (263)	228 (248)	195 (215)
		Exact	276	270	264	247	214
0.95	0.80	Chi-square	99 (112)	96 (109)	94 (107)	88 (101)	76 (89)
		Arcsine	91 (104)	89 (102)	87 (100)	81 (94)	70 (83)
		Exact	104	102	99	94	82

The values in parentheses are the sample size per group by the corresponding method with CC

tested at the significance level of $\alpha = 0.025$ by a one-sided test. We use the correlation coefficient of the multivariate Bernoulli distribution to define the associations among endpoints, assuming $\tau_T^{kk'} = \tau_C^{kk'} = \tau^{kk'}$, because it is intuitively attractive. In the exact method, 1,000,000 data sets are generated to evaluate the power.

Tables 3.2, 3.3 and 3.4 provide the equal sample sizes per group $n = n_T = n_C$ (i.e., $r = 1.0$) for two endpoints ($K = 2$) with correlation $\tau^{12} = 0.0$ (no correlation), 0.3 (low correlation), 0.5 (moderate correlation), 0.8 (high correlation), and 1.0 (perfect correlation), when $\pi_{T1} = \pi_{T2}$ and $\pi_{C1} = \pi_{C2}$.

Table 3.5 Sample size per group ($n = n_T = n_C$, $r = 1.0$) for three endpoints ($K = 3$) with the overall power of $1 - \beta = 0.80$

Proportions		Method	Correlations $\tau^{12} = \tau^{13} = \tau^{23}$				
π_{Tk}	π_{Ck}		0.0	0.3	0.5	0.8	1.0
0.55	0.50	Chi-square	2336 (2376)	2253 (2293)	2169 (2209)	1968 (2007)	1565 (1605)
		Arcsine	2337 (2376)	2254 (2294)	2169 (2209)	1968 (2008)	1565 (1605)
		Exact	2378	2299	2220	2018	1606
0.60	0.50	Chi-square	578 (598)	558 (578)	537 (557)	487 (507)	388 (408)
		Arcsine	579 (598)	558 (578)	537 (557)	487 (507)	388 (407)
		Exact	596	582	556	512	404
0.65	0.50	Chi-square	253 (266)	244 (257)	235 (248)	213 (226)	170 (184)
		Arcsine	253 (266)	244 (257)	235 (248)	213 (226)	170 (183)
		Exact	267	253	248	225	183
0.70	0.50	Chi-square	139 (148)	134 (144)	129 (139)	117 (127)	93 (103)
		Arcsine	139 (149)	134 (144)	129 (139)	117 (127)	93 (103)
		Exact	148	144	137	127	102
0.75	0.50	Chi-square	86 (94)	83 (91)	80 (88)	73 (80)	58 (66)
		Arcsine	86 (94)	83 (91)	80 (88)	72 (80)	58 (66)
		Exact	93	90	87	79	64
0.80	0.50	Chi-square	57 (64)	55 (62)	53 (60)	49 (55)	39 (46)
		Arcsine	57 (64)	55 (62)	53 (59)	48 (55)	38 (45)
		Exact	63	62	59	54	44
0.85	0.50	Chi-square	40 (45)	39 (44)	37 (43)	34 (39)	27 (33)
		Arcsine	39 (45)	38 (44)	37 (42)	33 (39)	27 (32)
		Exact	45	43	42	38	32
0.90	0.50	Chi-square	29 (33)	28 (33)	27 (32)	24 (29)	20 (25)
		Arcsine	28 (32)	27 (31)	26 (31)	23 (28)	19 (24)
		Exact	32	31	30	28	23
0.95	0.50	Chi-square	21 (25)	20 (25)	20 (24)	18 (22)	15 (20)
		Arcsine	19 (23)	19 (23)	18 (22)	16 (20)	13 (17)
		Exact	23	22	21	20	17

The values in parentheses are the sample size per group by the corresponding method with CC

Similarly as seen in multiple continuous endpoints, when $\pi_{T1} = \pi_{T2}$ and $\pi_{C1} = \pi_{C2}$, i.e., the standardized effect size $(\pi_{Tk} - \pi_{Ck})/\sqrt{\pi_{Tk}\theta_{Tk} + \pi_{Ck}\theta_{Ck}}$ are equal between two endpoints, the sample size decreases as the correlation approaches one. Comparing the cases of $\tau^{12} = 0.0$ and $\tau^{12} = 0.8$, the decrease in the sample size is approximately 11 %. Therefore, there is an advantage of incorporating the correlation among endpoints into the power and sample size calculations with co-primary binary endpoints.

Table 3.6 Sample size per group ($n = n_T = n_C$, $r = 1.0$) for three endpoints ($K = 3$) with the overall power of $1 - \beta = 0.80$

Proportions		Method	Correlations $\tau^{12} = \tau^{13} = \tau^{23}$				
π_{Tk}	π_{Ck}		0.0	0.3	0.5	0.8	1.0
0.65	0.60	Chi-square	2195 (2235)	2118 (2158)	2038 (2078)	1849 (1889)	1471 (1511)
		Arcsine	2196 (2235)	2118 (2158)	2039 (2078)	1849 (1889)	1471 (1510)
		Exact	2236	2161	2084	1892	1514
0.70	0.60	Chi-square	531 (551)	512 (532)	493 (513)	448 (467)	356 (376)
		Arcsine	531 (551)	512 (532)	493 (513)	447 (467)	356 (376)
		Exact	551	531	512	466	375
0.75	0.60	Chi-square	227 (240)	219 (232)	210 (224)	191 (204)	152 (166)
		Arcsine	226 (239)	218 (231)	210 (223)	191 (204)	152 (165)
		Exact	239	230	223	203	164
0.80	0.60	Chi-square	121 (131)	117 (127)	113 (122)	102 (112)	82 (92)
		Arcsine	120 (130)	116 (126)	112 (122)	101 (111)	81 (91)
		Exact	130	125	121	111	90
0.85	0.60	Chi-square	73 (81)	70 (78)	68 (75)	62 (69)	49 (57)
		Arcsine	72 (79)	69 (77)	67 (74)	60 (68)	48 (56)
		Exact	78	76	74	68	56
0.90	0.60	Chi-square	47 (53)	45 (52)	44 (50)	40 (46)	32 (39)
		Arcsine	45 (51)	43 (50)	42 (48)	38 (44)	30 (37)
		Exact	51	49	48	45	36
0.95	0.60	Chi-square	31 (37)	30 (36)	29 (35)	27 (32)	22 (28)
		Arcsine	28 (34)	27 (33)	26 (32)	24 (29)	19 (25)
		Exact	34	32	32	30	24

The values in parentheses are the sample size per group by the corresponding method with CC

Although the results are not shown here, when the standardized effect size for one endpoint is relatively smaller than that for other endpoints, the sample size does not change considerably as the correlation varies. In such cases, the advantage of incorporating the correlation into sample size is minimal. The power and sample size are more affected by the smaller standardized effect sizes than the correlation.

Similar to the case of two endpoints, Tables 3.5, 3.6 and 3.7 provide the equal sample sizes per group $n = n_T = n_C$ (i.e., $r = 1.0$) for three endpoints ($K = 3$) when $\pi_{T1} = \pi_{T2} = \pi_{T3}$ and $\pi_{C1} = \pi_{C2} = \pi_{C3}$, where the off-diagonal elements of the correlation matrix are equal, i.e., $\tau = \tau^{12} = \tau^{13} = \tau^{23} = 0.0, 0.3, 0.5, 0.8$, and 1.0. Comparing the cases of $\tau = 0.0$ and $\tau = 0.8$, the decrease in the sample size is approximately 16%. There is a larger relative efficiency with incorporation of correlation into trial sizing with more endpoints.

Table 3.7 Sample size per group ($n = n_T = n_C, r = 1.0$) for three endpoints ($K = 3$) with the overall power of $1 - \beta = 0.80$

Proportions		Method	Correlations $\tau^{12} = \tau^{13} = \tau^{23}$				
π_{Tk}	π_{Ck}		0.0	0.3	0.5	0.8	1.0
0.75	0.70	Chi-square	1867 (1907)	1801 (1841)	1734 (1774)	1573 (1613)	1251 (1291)
		Arcsine	1866 (1906)	1800 (1840)	1733 (1773)	1572 (1612)	1250 (1290)
		Exact	1908	1840	1771	1610	1292
0.80	0.70	Chi-square	437 (457)	422 (442)	406 (426)	369 (388)	294 (314)
		Arcsine	436 (456)	421 (440)	405 (425)	367 (387)	292 (312)
		Exact	456	439	425	387	311
0.85	0.70	Chi-square	180 (193)	173 (186)	167 (180)	152 (165)	121 (135)
		Arcsine	178 (191)	171 (184)	165 (178)	150 (163)	119 (132)
		Exact	190	184	177	162	131
0.90	0.70	Chi-square	92 (101)	89 (98)	85 (95)	78 (87)	62 (72)
		Arcsine	89 (98)	85 (95)	82 (92)	75 (84)	60 (69)
		Exact	98	94	91	85	69
0.95	0.70	Chi-square	52 (60)	50 (58)	49 (56)	44 (52)	36 (44)
		Arcsine	47 (55)	46 (53)	44 (52)	40 (48)	32 (40)
		Exact	55	53	52	48	39
0.85	0.80	Chi-square	1352 (1391)	1304 (1344)	1255 (1295)	1139 (1178)	906 (946)
		Arcsine	1348 (1388)	1300 (1340)	1251 (1291)	1135 (1175)	903 (942)
		Exact	1387	1340	1291	1174	942
0.90	0.80	Chi-square	297 (317)	286 (306)	276 (295)	250 (270)	199 (219)
		Arcsine	292 (311)	281 (301)	271 (290)	246 (265)	195 (215)
		Exact	309	301	290	266	214
0.95	0.80	Chi-square	112 (125)	108 (121)	104 (117)	95 (107)	76 (89)
		Arcsine	104 (117)	100 (113)	96 (109)	88 (101)	70 (83)
		Exact	118	114	109	100	82

The values in parentheses are the sample size per group by the corresponding method with CC

3.4 Example

We illustrate the sample size calculation methods with an application to the clinical trial (Ho et al. 2008); a randomized, parallel-treatment, placebo-controlled, double-blind, multicenter trial evaluating interventions for migraine headaches. Although, the trial has four interventions: (1) oral telcagepant 150 mg (low-dose), (2) oral telcagepant 300 mg (high-dose), (3), zolmitriptan 5 mg, and (4) placebo, and five co-primary endpoints: (1) pain freedom, (2) pain relief, (3) photophobia, (4) phonophobia, and (5) nausea, we consider a two-group comparison between the high-dose

Table 3.8 Equal sample size per group required to detect the superiority for all of the endpoints with the overall power of $1 - \beta = 0.80$ for a one-sided test at the significance level of $\alpha = 0.025$

	Method	Correlations ($\tau^{12}\ \tau^{13}\ \tau^{23}$)						
		000	00L	00M	00H	LLL	LLM	LLH
Empirical power	Chi-square	120	118	117	113	116	114	111
	Chi-square test	0.806	0.808	0.822	0.814	0.818	0.814	0.813
	Fisher's exact test	0.752	0.757	0.771	0.765	0.770	0.767	0.764
Empirical power	Chi-square with CC	130	128	127	123	126	124	120
	Chi-square test	0.815	0.810	0.811	0.806	0.809	0.807	0.800
	Fisher's exact test	0.815	0.810	0.811	0.806	0.809	0.807	0.801
Empirical power	Arcsine	119	117	116	112	115	113	109
	Chi-square test	0.808	0.814	0.815	0.807	0.813	0.808	0.805
	Fisher's exact test	0.749	0.761	0.764	0.756	0.764	0.757	0.751
Empirical power	Arcsine with CC	129	127	125	122	125	123	119
	Chi-square test	0.811	0.803	0.804	0.806	0.803	0.801	0.806
	Fisher's exact test	0.811	0.803	0.804	0.802	0.803	0.800	0.802
	Exact	128	127	126	122	125	123	117

Value of correlations: L = 0.3, M = 0.5, H = 0.8

group and the placebo group using three co-primary endpoints of pain freedom ($k = 1$), phonophobia ($k = 2$), and photophobia ($k = 3$). From the results of the trial (for details, see Table 3.4 in Ho et al. 2008), the response probability for each endpoint is assumed to be $(\pi_{T1}, \pi_{T2}, \pi_{T3}) = (0.269, 0.578, 0.510)$ for the high-dose group and $(\pi_{C1}, \pi_{C2}, \pi_{C3}) = (0.096, 0.368, 0.289)$ for the placebo group. Under these values, the ranges for the correlation coefficient $\tau_T^{kk'}$ and $\tau_C^{kk'}$ are given by

$$\text{Pain freedom} \quad -0.71 \le \tau_T^{12} \le 0.52 \quad -0.25 \le \tau_C^{12} \le 0.43$$
$$\text{Phonophobia} \quad -0.62 \le \tau_T^{13} \le 0.59 \quad -0.23 \le \tau_C^{13} \le 0.47$$
$$\text{Photophobia} \quad -0.84 \le \tau_T^{23} \le 0.87 \quad -0.53 \le \tau_C^{23} \le 0.91.$$

Furthermore, under the situation of $\tau_T^{kk'} = \tau_C^{kk'} = \tau^{kk'}$ the ranges are given by

$$\max(-0.71, -0.25) = -0.25 \le \tau^{12} \le \min(0.52, 0.43) = 0.43$$
$$\max(-0.62, -0.23) = -0.23 \le \tau^{13} \le \min(0.59, 0.47) = 0.47$$
$$\max(-0.84, -0.53) = -0.53 \le \tau^{23} \le \min(0.87, 0.91) = 0.87.$$

Table 3.8 presents the required equal sample sizes per group $n = n_T = n_C$ (i.e., $r = 1.0$) with the overall power of $1 - \beta = 0.80$ for $(\delta_1, \delta_2, \delta_3) = (0.173, 0.210, 0.221)$ at the significance level of $\alpha = 0.025$, where $\tau^{12} = \tau^{13} \le \tau^{23}$. The empirical (overall) power for the chi-square and Fisher's exact tests was calculated under the given sample size with 100,000 Monte-Carlo trials. In this setting, the sample size decreases by about 8 %, when considering the correlations among the endpoints compared to a naive calculation that assumes zero correlation.

3.5 Summary

This chapter provides methods for power and sample size determination for clinical trials with an alternative hypothesis of joint differences in proportions when all of the endpoints are binary variables. We evaluated the behaviors of the sample sizes and empirical powers presented in Appendix B for the methods using the chi-square and arcsine methods with and without CC, and the exact method. Our major findings are as follows:

- Similarly as seen with multiple continuous endpoints, there is an advantage of incorporating the correlation among endpoints into the power and sample size calculations with co-primary binary endpoints as the power is improved and the sample size is decreased relative to naive calculations assuming zero correlation. Relative efficiency is greater as the number of endpoints increases. When the endpoints are positively correlated (correlation up to 0.8) and the standardized effect sizes among endpoints are approximately equal, there is approximately 11 % reduction in the case of two co-primary endpoints and 16 % reduction in the case of three co-primary endpoints. When the standardized effect size for one endpoint is relatively smaller than that for other endpoints, the advantage of incorporating the correlation into sample size is minimal as the power and sample size are primarily affected by the standardized effect size than the correlation.
- The chi-square method (without CC) works well in most situations except for extremely small sample sizes (i.e., the extremely large difference in two proportions): the empirical power for the method achieves the targeted power when the difference in proportions is not extremely large. In other situations, the empirical power tends to be larger than the targeted power. The arcsine method with CC leads to sample sizes approximately equal to those obtained by the exact method. Recently, Lydersen et al. (2009) discussed the choice of testing methods for a sigle primary endpoint in 2×2 tables.
- The choice of an association measure may depend on several factors including the nature and characteristics of endpoints and the statistical methods used for data analysis. However, as the number of endpoints increases, the added complexity can affect the sample size determination. This leads to a non-negligible, practical, challenge regarding the specification of the values of the association measures because the increased number of endpoints imposes greater range restrictions on the association measures. It is difficult to precisely determine all of the values from the data. This implies that researchers should be extremely careful when considering the selection of numerous primary endpoints. Therefore, we generally recommend selection of a minimal number of primary endpoints that directly relate to the primary objective.

References

Bartlett MS (1947) The use of transformations. Biometrics 3:39–52

Emrich LJ, Piedmonte MR (1991) A method for generating high-dimensional multivariate binary variates. Am Stat 45:302–304

Ho TW, Ferrari MD, Dodick DW, Galet V, Kost J, Fan X, Leibensperger H, Froman S, Assaid C, Lines C, Koppen H, Winner PK (2008) Efficacy and tolerability of MK-0974 (telcagepant), a new oral antagonist of calcitonin gene-related peptide receptor, compared with zolmitriptan for acute migraine: a randomised, placebo-controlled, parallel-treatment trial. Lancet 37:2115–2123

Johnson NL, Kotz S, Balakrishnan N (1997) Discrete multivariate distributions. Wiley, New York

Lydersen S, Fagerland MW, Laake P (2009) Recommended tests for association in 2×2 tables. Stat Med 28:1159–1175

Pearson K (1900) On the criterion that a given system of deviations from the probable in the case of a correlated system of variables is such that it can be reasonably supposed to have arisen from random sampling. Philos Mag Ser B 50:157–175

Prentice RL (1988) Correlated binary regression with covariates specific to each binary observarion. Biometrics 44:1033–1048

Sozu T, Sugimoto T, Hamasaki T (2010) Sample size determination in clinical trials with multiple co-primary binary endpoints. Stat Med 29:2169–2179

Sozu T, Sugimoto T, Hamasaki T (2011) Sample size determination in superiority clinical trials with multiple co-primary correlated endpoints. J Biopharm Stat 21:650–668

Walters DE (1979) In defence of the arc sine approximation. Statistician 28:219–222

Yates F (1934) Contingency tables involving small numbers and the χ^2 test. J Roy. Stat Soc Supplement. 1:217–235

Chapter 4
Convenient Sample Size Formula

Abstract In Chaps. 2 and 3, we discuss the methods for calculating the sample size required to design a trial with multiple co-primary endpoints. These methods require considerable mathematical sophistication and knowledge of programming techniques, effectively limiting their application in practice. To increase the practicality of these methods, in this chapter we provide an efficient algorithm for calculating the sample size and present a convenient sample size formula with associated numerical tables for sizing clinical trials with multiple co-primary endpoints. We provide numerical examples to illustrate use of the formula and associated tables, and provide the programming codes for the R and SAS software packages.

Keywords Newton-Raphson algorithm · Numerical table · R · SAS

4.1 Introduction

An iterative procedure is required to find the sample size that achieves the desired overall power using the methods discussed in Chaps. 2 and 3. The easiest method involves a grid search to increase n gradually until the power exceeds the desired overall power. However, this method requires mathematical sophistication, specialized programming knowledge, and often takes considerable computing time.

In this chapter we provide an efficient and practical algorithm for calculating the sample size and present a practical sample size formula with associated numerical tables for sizing clinical trials with multiple co-primary endpoints. The formula reduces to a very familiar one if the number of primary endpoints is one. The formula and associated tables have the following advantages: (i) they are easy to use, are convenient, inexpensive, and practical; (ii) they provide intuition regarding the relationship between factors such as type I and II errors, effect sizes, correlation, and variance, revealing how these factors affect the required sample size; and (iii) they allow for an informative graphical display that is helpful in evaluating the sample size sensitivity.

© The Author(s) 2015

T. Sozu et al., *Sample Size Determination in Clinical Trials with Multiple Endpoints*, SpringerBriefs in Statistics, DOI 10.1007/978-3-319-22005-5_4

4.2 Convenient Formula

4.2.1 Continuous Endpoints

Consider a randomized clinical trial comparing two interventions with n_T subjects in the test group and n_C subjects in the control group. There are K co-primary continuous endpoints with a K-variate normal distribution, where $K \geq 2$. Let the responses for the n_T subjects in the test group be denoted by Y_{Tjk}, $j = 1, \ldots, n_T$, and those for the n_C subjects in the control group, by Y_{Cjk}, $j = 1, \ldots, n_C$. Suppose that the vectors of responses $\boldsymbol{Y}_{Tj} = (Y_{Tj1}, \ldots, Y_{TjK})^T$ and $\boldsymbol{Y}_{Cj} = (Y_{Cj1}, \ldots, Y_{CjK})^T$ are independently distributed as K-variate normal distributions with mean vectors $E[\boldsymbol{Y}_{Tj}] = \boldsymbol{\mu}_T = (\mu_{T1}, \ldots, \mu_{TK})^T$ and $E[\boldsymbol{Y}_{Cj}] = \boldsymbol{\mu}_C = (\mu_{C1}, \ldots, \mu_{CK})^T$, respectively, and common covariance matrix $\boldsymbol{\Sigma}$, i.e.,

$$\boldsymbol{Y}_{Tj} \sim N_K(\boldsymbol{\mu}_T, \boldsymbol{\Sigma}) \quad \text{and} \quad \boldsymbol{Y}_{Cj} \sim N_K(\boldsymbol{\mu}_C, \boldsymbol{\Sigma}),$$

where

$$\boldsymbol{\Sigma} = \begin{pmatrix} \sigma_1^2 & \cdots & \rho^{1K}\sigma_1\sigma_K \\ \vdots & \ddots & \vdots \\ \rho^{1K}\sigma_1\sigma_K & \cdots & \sigma_K^2 \end{pmatrix}$$

with $\mathrm{var}[Y_{Tjk}] = \mathrm{var}[Y_{Cjk}] = \sigma_k^2$, $\mathrm{corr}[Y_{Tjk}, Y_{Tjk'}] = \mathrm{corr}[Y_{Cjk}, Y_{Cjk'}] = \rho^{kk'}$ $(k \neq k' : 1 \leq k < k' \leq K)$.

We can assert the superiority of the test intervention over the control in terms of all K primary endpoints if and only if $\mu_{Tk} - \mu_{Ck} > 0$ for all $k = 1, \ldots, K$. Thus, the hypotheses for testing are

$$\begin{aligned} &H_0 : \mu_{Tk} - \mu_{Ck} \leq 0 \text{ for at least one } k, \\ &H_1 : \mu_{Tk} - \mu_{Ck} > 0 \text{ for all k.} \end{aligned} \tag{4.1}$$

In testing the preceding hypotheses, the null hypothesis H_0 is rejected if and only if all of the null hypotheses associated with each of the K primary endpoints are rejected at a significance level of α.

Similarly as in Sect. 2.2.1, under the assumption that the variance is known, the following Z-statistic can be used to test the difference in the means for each endpoint:

$$Z_k = \frac{\bar{Y}_{Tk} - \bar{Y}_{Ck}}{\sigma_k\sqrt{\dfrac{1}{n_T} + \dfrac{1}{n_C}}}, \quad k = 1, \ldots, K, \tag{4.2}$$

where $\bar{Y}_{Tk}$ and $\bar{Y}_{Ck}$ are the sample means given by

$$\bar{Y}_{Tk} = \frac{1}{n_T} \sum_{j=1}^{n_T} Y_{Tjk} \quad \text{and} \quad \bar{Y}_{Ck} = \frac{1}{n_C} \sum_{j=1}^{n_C} Y_{Cjk}.$$

Hence, the sample size required for achieving the desired power of $1 - \beta$ is obtained by the minimum n that satisfies

$$1 - \beta \leq \int_{z_\alpha}^{\infty} \cdots \int_{z_\alpha}^{\infty} f_{\rho_Z}(z_1, \ldots, z_K; \sqrt{n\kappa}\delta) dz_K \cdots dz_1, \qquad (4.3)$$

where $r = n_C/n_T$, $n = n_T$, $\kappa = r/(1+r)$, $\delta = (\delta_1, \ldots, \delta_K)^T$, $\delta_k = (\mu_{Tk} - \mu_{Ck})/\sigma_k$ (standardized effect size), and $f_{\rho_Z}(\cdot; m)$ is the density function of the multivariate normal (MVN) with mean vector m and correlation matrix ρ_Z. The off-diagonal elements of ρ_Z is given by $\rho^{kk'}$. Further, z_α is the $(1 - \alpha)$ quantile of the standard normal distribution. An algorithm that can be used to obtain such an n involves evaluating (4.3) in which n is replaced with $\tilde{n} \leftarrow \tilde{n} + 1$ being updated consecutively from a starting point n_0 for $\tilde{n}$. As the starting point, we can use

$$n_0 = \frac{(z_\beta + z_\alpha)^2}{\kappa \cdot \min_k \delta_k^2}, \qquad (4.4)$$

i.e., the sample size per group required in the case of a single endpoint with the minimum effect size, where z_β is the $(1 - \beta)$ quantile of the standard normal distribution.

Example 1 Consider the case of $\delta_1 = 0.55$ and $\delta_2 = 0.50$ with the equal sample sizes per group $n = n_T = n_C$ (i.e., $r = 1.0$), $\rho^{12} = 0.5$ and $\alpha = 0.025$. Starting points of $n_0 = 62.8$ and 84.1 are computed in advance for $1 - \beta = 0.8$ and 0.9, respectively. Table 4.1 displays the computational processes for $(\tilde{n}, n)$ and the corresponding power updated consecutively until (4.3) is achieved.

Although it may appear computationally simple to evaluate (4.3) when there are two endpoints, the computation requires an iterative algorithm equipped with the cumulative distribution function (CDF) of the MVN. Computation is more complicated when there are three or more endpoints. Thus, we provide a simple formula

Table 4.1 Computational processes for $(\tilde{n}, n)$ and the corresponding power until (4.3) is satisfied under the equal sample sizes per group $n = n_T = n_C$ (i.e., $r = 1.0$), $\delta_1 = 0.55$, $\delta_2 = 0.50$, $\rho^{12} = 0.5$ and $\alpha = 0.025$

$\tilde{n}$	$[n_0]$ 63	64	65	66	67	68	69	70	71	72 $[n]$
Power	0.734	0.742	0.750	0.758	0.765	0.773	0.780	0.787	0.794	0.800
$\tilde{n}$	$[n_0]$ 85	86	87	88	89	90	91	92	93 $[n]$	
Power	0.871	0.875	0.879	0.883	0.888	0.891	0.895	0.899	0.902	

expressed as "$n =$" for practical use, which researchers can use to calculate the sample size as easily as if there were a single endpoint.

An alternative formula for (4.3) is

$$n = \frac{(C_K + z_\alpha)^2}{\kappa \cdot \delta_K^2} \tag{4.5}$$

using C_K which is the solution of the integral equation

$$1 - \beta = \int_{-\infty}^{\gamma_1 C_K + z_\alpha(\gamma_1 - 1)} \cdots \int_{-\infty}^{\gamma_{K-1} C_K + z_\alpha(\gamma_{K-1} - 1)} \int_{-\infty}^{C_K} f_{\rho_Z}(z_1, \ldots, z_K; \mathbf{0}) dz_K \cdots dz_1, \tag{4.6}$$

where the γ_k terms are the effect size ratios given by $\gamma_k = \delta_k/\delta_K$ for $k = 1, \ldots, K-1$. It is appropriate to write $C_K = C_K(\beta, \boldsymbol{\rho}_Z, \boldsymbol{\gamma}, \alpha)$ in the formal manner because the solution of (4.6) for C_K depends on β, $\boldsymbol{\rho}_Z$, $\boldsymbol{\gamma}$ and α, where $\boldsymbol{\gamma} = (\gamma_1, \ldots, \gamma_{K-1})$. The C_K term in (4.5) corresponds to z_β in the sample size formula in the case of the single endpoint. In fact, C_K reduces to z_β if $K = 1$. Because users are familiar with the univariate sample size formula, (4.5) may be more appealing than (4.3). Users can calculate the required sample size per group by providing C_K from the tables or from an algorithm as discussed later. In addition, formula (4.5) reveals how the sample size is influenced by factors such as type I and II errors, effect sizes and correlation. For example, the ratio of $n(\rho)$ to $n(0)$ is easily derived from (4.5). In particular, if effect sizes are the same for each endpoint under a common α and β, then the ratio is determined depending only on C_K which varies with the correlation matrix $\boldsymbol{\rho}_Z$, that is,

$$\frac{n(\rho)}{n(0)} = \frac{(C_K(\beta, \boldsymbol{\rho}_Z, \boldsymbol{\gamma}, \alpha) + z_\alpha)^2}{(C_K(\beta, \mathbf{I}, \boldsymbol{\gamma}, \alpha) + z_\alpha)^2},$$

where $n(0)$ is the sample sizes per group required in the uncorrelated case and $\mathbf{I}$ is the identity matrix. This result could not be determined using (4.3). In Fig. 4.1, we provide plots of the ratio $(n(\rho)/n(0))$ against ρ^{12} for $K = 2$, $\alpha = 0.025$ and $\beta = 0.2$ when the effect size ratios are $\gamma_1 = 1.0, 1.1, 1.2, 1.3, 1.4, 1.5$ and 2.0. For example, the ratio is about 89 % when $\rho^{12} = 0.8$ and $\gamma_1 = 1.0$, which agrees with a discussion of Sozu et al. (2011) and Fig. 2.4 in Sect. 2.4.3. Figure 4.1 shows that the ratio decreases as the correlation approaches one. Even when $\gamma_1 > 1.0$, the ratio still decreases as the correlation approaches one. However, when $\gamma_1 > 1.5$, the ratio does not change considerably as the correlation varies. In addition, the larger K is, the more remarkably the ratio changes with the correlation matrix $\boldsymbol{\rho}_Z$.

Now we show how (4.5) is derived from (4.3). By shifting the density function to $-\sqrt{n\kappa}\boldsymbol{\delta}$ and using the symmetry property on the domain of integration, we can transform the equation version of (4.3) into

$$1 - \beta = \int_{-\infty}^{\sqrt{n\kappa}\delta_1 - z_\alpha} \cdots \int_{-\infty}^{\sqrt{n\kappa}\delta_K - z_\alpha} f_{\rho_Z}(z_1, \ldots, z_K; \mathbf{0}) dz_K \cdots dz_1,$$

where $\mathbf{0} = (0, \ldots, 0)^T$. This equation is equivalent to the simultaneous equations

$$1 - \beta = \int_{-\infty}^{C_1} \cdots \int_{-\infty}^{C_K} f_{\rho_Z}(z_1, \ldots, z_K; \mathbf{0}) dz_K \cdots dz_1, \qquad (4.7a)$$

$$\text{and} \quad C_k = \sqrt{n\kappa}\delta_k - z_\alpha, k = 1, \ldots, K. \qquad (4.7b)$$

Note that (4.7b) is equivalent to K linear equations

$$\begin{cases} n = \kappa^{-1}(C_1 + z_\alpha)^2/\delta_1^2, \\ \qquad \vdots \\ n = \kappa^{-1}(C_K + z_\alpha)^2/\delta_K^2. \end{cases} \qquad (4.7c)$$

Considering a combination of (4.7a), (4.7b) and (4.7c), we can derive a formula for n, such as (4.5). For example, given C_K (one of the C_k terms), the remaining C_k terms are expressed as

$$C_k = \gamma_k C_K + z_\alpha (\gamma_k - 1), \quad k = 1, \ldots, K - 1 \qquad (4.8)$$

using $(K - 1)$ equations of (4.7b) or (4.7c). Then, the integral equation (4.6) is obtained by substituting (4.8) into (4.7a). Therefore, using the solution of (4.6) for C_K, we have (4.5) represented by the form of "$n =$". In summary, (4.5) is a transformation equivalent to the equation version of (4.3), which is the sample size formula to achieve the power of $1 - \beta$ when there are K co-primary endpoints. We provide the numerical values of C_k for $K = 2$ in Tables 4.3 and 4.4, and $K = 3$ in Tables C.1 and C.2 in Appendix C.

Fig. 4.1 Behavior of the ratio $(n(\rho)/n(0))$ for $K = 2$, $\alpha = 0.025$ and $\beta = 0.2$ under $\gamma_1 = 1.0, 1.1, 1.2, 1.3, 1.4, 1.5$ and 2.0

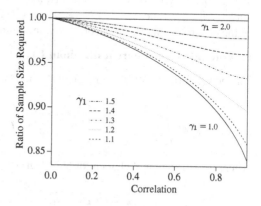

4.2.2 Binary Endpoints

For K co-primary binary endpoints, Chap. 3 provided the formulae for power and sample size calculation in a two-group comparison using five testing methods (the chi-square and arcsine methods with and without CC, and the exact method). Here, we show how the formula (4.5) for continuous co-primary endpoints is modified for binary endpoints, in particular when the testing methods except for the exact method are used.

In this section, suppose that the vector of responses Y_{Tj}, $j = 1, \ldots, n_T$ and Y_{Cj}, $j = 1, \ldots, n_C$ are independently distributed as K-variate Bernoulli distribution with means $\mu_{Tk} = E[Y_{Tjk}] = \pi_{Tk}$ and $\mu_{Ck} = E[Y_{Cjk}] = \pi_{Ck}$ and correlations (of binary endpoints)

$$\tau_T^{kk'} = \frac{\phi_T^{kk'} - \pi_{Tk}\pi_{Tk'}}{\sqrt{\pi_{Tk}\theta_{Tk}\pi_{Tk'}\theta_{Tk'}}} \quad \text{and} \quad \tau_C^{kk'} = \frac{\phi_C^{kk'} - \pi_{Ck}\pi_{Ck'}}{\sqrt{\pi_{Ck}\theta_{Ck}\pi_{Ck'}\theta_{Ck'}}},$$

where $\phi_T^{kk'} = \Pr[Y_{Tjk} = Y_{Tjk'} = 1]$, $\phi_C^{kk'} = \Pr[Y_{Cjk} = Y_{Cjk'} = 1]$, $\theta_{Tk} = 1 - \pi_{Tk}$, and $\theta_{Ck} = 1 - \pi_{Ck}$. We write $n_T = n$ and $n_C = nr$ using the ratio $r = n_C/n_T$, and denote $\kappa = r/(1 + r)$. Throughout the paragraph of the chi-square methods below, denote $\delta_k = (\pi_{Tk} - \pi_{Ck})/\sigma_k$ and

$$\begin{cases} \sigma_k = \sqrt{\dfrac{\kappa\pi_{Tk}\theta_{Tk} + (1 - \kappa)\pi_{Ck}\theta_{Ck}}{\kappa}} \\[4mm] \sigma_k^* = \sqrt{\dfrac{((1 - \kappa)\pi_{Tk} + \kappa\pi_{Ck})((1 - \kappa)\theta_{Tk} + \kappa\theta_{Ck})}{\kappa}} \end{cases}, \quad k = 1, \ldots, K.$$

While, in the part of the arcsine methods, we will use $\delta_k = (\sin^{-1}\sqrt{\pi_{Tk}} - \sin^{-1}\sqrt{\pi_{Ck}})/\sigma_k$ and $\sigma_k = 1/2\sqrt{\kappa}$, $k = 1, \ldots, K$. See Table 3.1 for the details of the covariance matrix ρ_{Z*} corresponding to these four methods.

(1) One-sided chi-square test without CC (Pearson 1900)

The power formula for the chi-square method (without CC) is provided by

$$1 - \beta \simeq \int_{-\infty}^{\sqrt{n}\delta_1 - \frac{\sigma_1^*}{\sigma_1}z_\alpha} \cdots \int_{-\infty}^{\sqrt{n}\delta_K - \frac{\sigma_K^*}{\sigma_K}z_\alpha} f_{\rho_{Z*}}(z_1, \ldots, z_K; \mathbf{0})dz_K \cdots dz_1,$$

where the off-diagonal element of the covariance matrix ρ_{Z*} is

$$\rho_D^{kk'} = \frac{\kappa\tau_T^{kk'}\sqrt{\pi_{Tk}\theta_{Tk}\pi_{Tk'}\theta_{Tk'}} + (1 - \kappa)\tau_C^{kk'}\sqrt{\pi_{Ck}\theta_{Ck}\pi_{Ck'}\theta_{Ck'}}}{\kappa\sigma_k\sigma_{k'}}.$$

Let $C_k = \sqrt{n}\delta_k - \dfrac{\sigma_k^*}{\sigma_k}z_\alpha$, then, similarly to the manner to derive (4.5), we have

$$n = \delta_k^{-2} \left(C_k + \frac{\sigma_k^*}{\sigma_k} z_\alpha \right)^2, \quad k = 1, \ldots, K.$$

So, given C_K, the rest C_k's are expressed by

$$C_k = \gamma_k C_K + z_\alpha \left(\frac{\sigma_K^*}{\sigma_K} \gamma_k - \frac{\sigma_k^*}{\sigma_k} \right). \tag{4.9}$$

where $\gamma_k = \delta_k / \delta_K, k = 1, \ldots, K - 1$. Hence, the sample size formula is

$$n = \frac{\left(C_K + \frac{\sigma_K^*}{\sigma_K} z_\alpha \right)^2}{\delta_K^2} \tag{4.10}$$

using the solution C_K of the integral equation

$$1 - \beta = \int_{-\infty}^{\gamma_1 C_K + z_\alpha \left(\frac{\sigma_K^*}{\sigma_K} \gamma_1 - \frac{\sigma_1^*}{\sigma_1} \right)} \cdots \int_{-\infty}^{\gamma_{K-1} C_K + z_\alpha \left(\frac{\sigma_K^*}{\sigma_K} \gamma_{K-1} - \frac{\sigma_{K-1}^*}{\sigma_{K-1}} \right)}$$

$$\times \int_{-\infty}^{C_K} f_{\rho_{Z^*}} (z_1, \ldots, z_K; \mathbf{0}) \, dz_K \cdots dz_1. \tag{4.11}$$

(2) One-sided chi-square test with CC (Yates 1934)

Letting

$$C_k = \sqrt{n} \delta_k - \frac{\sigma_k^*}{\sigma_k} z_\alpha - \frac{1}{2n\kappa} \frac{\sqrt{n}}{\sigma_k} = \sqrt{n} \delta_k - \frac{\sigma_k^*}{\sigma_k} z_\alpha - \frac{1}{2\sqrt{n}\kappa \sigma_k},$$

the power formula for the chi-square method with CC is provided similarly to the chi-square method (without CC) by

$$1 - \beta \simeq \int_{-\infty}^{C_1} \cdots \int_{-\infty}^{C_{K-1}} \int_{-\infty}^{C_K} f_{\rho_{Z^*}} (z_1, \ldots, z_K; \mathbf{0}) \, dz_K \ldots dz_1. \tag{4.12}$$

The definition of $\rho_D^{kk'}$ is the same as that of the chi-square method. Hence, the relationship between C_k and δ_k is more complicated than the chi-square method,

$$\delta_k n - \left(\frac{\sigma_k^*}{\sigma_k} z_\alpha + C_k \right) \sqrt{n} - \frac{1}{2\kappa\sigma_k} = 0,$$

so that we have

$$\sqrt{n} = \frac{z_\alpha \sigma_k^* / \sigma_k + C_k + \sqrt{(z_\alpha \sigma_k^* / \sigma_k + C_k)^2 + 2\delta_k / \kappa \sigma_k}}{2\delta_k}, \quad k = 1, \ldots, K.$$

This yields the non-linear equation between C_k and C_K as follows:

$$\frac{\delta_K}{\delta_k} \left\{ z_\alpha \sigma_k^* / \sigma_k + C_k + \sqrt{(z_\alpha \sigma_k^* / \sigma_k + C_k)^2 + 2\delta_k / \kappa \sigma_k} \right\}$$
$$= z_\alpha \sigma_K^* / \sigma_K + C_K + \sqrt{(z_\alpha \sigma_K^* / \sigma_K + C_K)^2 + 2\delta_K / \kappa \sigma_K}. \qquad (4.13)$$

Therefore, the required sample size per group is

$$n = \frac{\left(z_\alpha \sigma_K^* / \sigma_K + C_K + \sqrt{(z_\alpha \sigma_K^* / \sigma_K + C_K)^2 + 2\delta_K / \kappa \sigma_K} \right)^2}{4\delta_K^2}$$

using the solution C_K of the integral equation (4.12) satisfying (4.13). To obtain the solution C_k of (4.13) for given C_K, an iteration method such as the Newton-Raphson (NR) method is required.

(3) Arcsine root transformation method without CC (Bartlett 1947)

Let $\delta_k = (\sin^{-1} \sqrt{\pi_{Tk}} - \sin^{-1} \sqrt{\pi_{Ck}}) / \sigma_k$ and $\sigma_k = 1/2\sqrt{\kappa}$, $k = 1, \ldots, K$. Then, because σ_k is independent of π_{Tk} and π_{Ck}, the power formula for the arcsine method (without CC) is the same as that for continuous endpoint in the previous section. Therefore, the sample size formula is

$$n = \frac{(C_K + z_\alpha)^2}{\delta_K^2} \qquad (4.14)$$

using the solution C_K of the integral equation

$$1 - \beta = \int_{-\infty}^{\gamma_1 C_K + z_\alpha(\gamma_1 - 1)} \cdots \int_{-\infty}^{\gamma_{K-1} C_K + z_\alpha(\gamma_{K-1} - 1)} \int_{-\infty}^{C_K} f_{\rho_{Z^*}}(z_1, \ldots, z_K; 0) \, dz_K \cdots dz_1,$$
$$(4.15)$$

where the (k, k')th element of the covariance matrix ρ_{Z^*} is $\rho_D^{kk'} = \kappa \tau_T^{kk'} + (1 - \kappa) \tau_C^{kk'}$ (see Sozu et al. 2010) and $\gamma_k = \delta_k / \delta_K$, $k = 1, \ldots, K - 1$. Note that (4.15) is the same as the Eq. (4.6) except the point that the covariance matrix ρ_{Z^*} is used instead of ρ_Z, so that the same algorithm to obtain C_K can be used in the both cases.

(4) Arcsine root transformation method with CC (Walters 1979)

In the arcsine method with CC, it is difficult to derive the form of "$n =$" as the sample size formula. This is because the correction terms of $(1 - \kappa)/2n\kappa$ as given in Table 3.1 appear not only in the square root of the arcsine function but also in the binomial variance forms. That is, the relationship between C_k and n is too complicated to express an explicit form of "$n =$", although it is linear in the chi-square and arcsine methods (without CC) and quadratic in the chi-square method with CC. Hence, a simple formula for the arcsine method with CC is not provided. An iterative procedure is required to find a required sample size. The sample size obtained from the arcsine method (without CC) can be used as an initial value in an algorithm for the sample size calculation.

4.3 Computational Algorithm

We provide an NR algorithm to solve (4.6), (4.11) and (4.15). Although the covariance matrix ρ is used throughout this section, the ρ is ρ_Z in the case of continuous endpoints and ρ_{Z*} in the case of binary endpoints. For simplicity, we consider the case of $K = 2$. Let

$$G(C_2) = (1 - \beta) - \int_{-\infty}^{\gamma_1 C_2 + z_\alpha (a_2 \gamma_1 - a_1)} \int_{-\infty}^{C_2} f_\rho(z_1, z_2; \mathbf{0}) \, dz_2 dz_1,$$

where $a_1 = \sigma_1^*/\sigma_1$ and $a_2 = \sigma_2^*/\sigma_2$ if the chi-square method (without CC) is used in the case of binary endpoints and $a_1 = a_2 = 1$ otherwise (see (4.9) and (4.8)). For the NR method, we need the first derivative of $G(C_2)$ in order to find $G(C_2) = 0$, which yields (4.6). The first derivative is

$$\frac{dG(C_2)}{dC_2} = -F_\rho^{(1)}(C_1, C_2)\gamma_1 - F_\rho^{(2)}(C_1, C_2),$$

where $C_1 = \gamma_1 C_2 + z_\alpha(a_2\gamma_1 - a_1)$ following (4.8) and (4.9),

$$F_\rho^{(1)}(C_1, C_2) = \int_{-\infty}^{C_2} f_\rho(C_1, z_2; \mathbf{0}) \, dz_2 \quad \text{and} \quad F_\rho^{(2)}(C_1, C_2) = \int_{-\infty}^{C_1} f_\rho(z_1, C_2; \mathbf{0}) \, dz_1.$$

Hence, we obtain the NR algorithm

$$C_2^{(l)} = C_2^{(l-1)} - \left\{ \frac{dG(C_2)}{dC_2} \right\}^{-1} G(C_2) \bigg|_{C_2 = C_2^{(l-1)}}, \quad l = 1, 2, \ldots,$$

where $C_2^{(0)}$ is the starting point of this algorithm. For example, as such a starting point, we can use z_β or the solution of $G(C_2) = 0$ when $\gamma_1 = 1$. In addition, $F_\rho^{(k)}$ can be computed approximately from the numerical derivative using the CDF of the MVN. Also, by a simple extension from $K = 2$, we obtain a general NR algorithm for solving the integral equation (4.6) for an arbitrary K. We describe these details generally in the following section.

Table 4.2 Newton-Raphson iterations of $C_2^{(l)}$ and the corresponding power and equal sample size per group $n^{(l)}$ ($r = 1.0$) when $\delta_1 = 0.55$, $\delta_2 = 0.50$, $\rho^{12} = 0.5$ and $\alpha = 0.025$

$\beta = 0.2$					$\beta = 0.1$				
l	0	1	2	3	l	0	1	2	3
$C_2^{(l)}$	0.8416	1.0248	1.0396	1.0397	$C_2^{(l)}$	1.2816	1.4226	1.4373	1.4374
Power	0.7326	0.7954	0.79997	0.8000	Power	0.8665	0.8971	0.89997	0.9000
$n^{(l)}$	62.79	71.27	71.98	71.98	$n^{(l)}$	84.06	91.53	92.33	92.34

Example 2 Consider the case in Example 1 (equal sample size per group $n = n_T = n_C$ (i.e., $r = 1.0$), $\delta_1 = 0.55$, $\delta_2 = 0.50$, $\rho^{12} = 0.5$ and $\alpha = 0.025$).

Because of the continuous endpoints, we use $a_1 = a_2 = 1$. In this case, the starting point, $C_2^{(0)}$ is z_β, which corresponds to selecting n_0. Table 4.2 shows two examples of a sequence for $C_2^{(l)}$, and the corresponding power and $n^{(l)}$ obtained from the NR iterations under $\beta = 0.2$ and $\beta = 0.1$, where $n^{(l)}$ is the n obtained from (4.5) in which C_K is replaced by $C_K^{(l)}$. In many cases, the NR algorithm completes the calculation using fewer iterations than is implied by the consecutive updating method for $(\tilde{n}, n)$ described in Example 1.

General Cases. Denote the CDF of the MVN with zero means by

$$F_\rho(C_1, \ldots, C_K) = \int_{-\infty}^{C_1} \cdots \int_{-\infty}^{C_K} f_\rho(z_1, \ldots, z_K; 0) dz_K \cdots dz_1.$$

In addition, denote the first partial derivative $\partial F_\rho(C_1, \ldots, C_K)/\partial C_k$ by $F_\rho^{(k)}(C_1, \ldots, C_K)$. Let

$$G(C_K) = (1 - \beta) - F_\rho(\gamma_1 C_K + z_\alpha(a_K \gamma_1 - a_1), \ldots, \gamma_{K-1} C_K + z_\alpha(a_K \gamma_{K-1} - a_{K-1}), C_K),$$

where $a_k = \sigma_k^*/\sigma_k$, $k = 1, 2, \ldots, K$ if the chi-square method (without CC) is used in the case of binary endpoints and $a_1 = a_2 = \cdots = a_K = 1$ otherwise (the cases of continuous endpoints and the arcsine method with CC). Note that (4.6) is the same as $G(C_K) = 0$. Then, a simple extension from the case of $K = 2$ gives the NR algorithm to solve (4.6) for an arbitrary K:

$$C_K^{(l)} = C_K^{(l-1)} - \left\{ \frac{dG(C_K)}{dC_K} \right\}^{-1} G(C_K) \Big|_{C_K = C_K^{(l-1)}}, \quad l = 1, 2, \ldots,$$

where these elements are evaluated by

$$\frac{dG(C_K)}{dC_K} = -\sum_{k=1}^{K-1} F_\rho^{(k)}(C_1, \ldots, C_K)\gamma_k - F_\rho^{(K)}(C_1, \ldots, C_K)$$

and $F_\rho^{(k)}(C_1, \ldots, C_K) = \int_{-\infty}^{C_1} \cdots \int_{-\infty}^{C_{k-1}} \int_{-\infty}^{C_{k+1}} \cdots \int_{-\infty}^{C_K}$
$$f_\rho(z_1, \ldots, z_{k-1}, C_k, z_{k+1}, \ldots, z_K) \, dz_K \cdots dz_{k+1} dz_{k-1} \cdots dz_1,$$

because $C_k = \gamma_k C_K + z_\alpha(a_K \gamma_k - a_k)$, $k = 1, \ldots, K - 1$ are given by (4.8) and (4.9). In many statistical software packages, $F_\rho^{(k)}$ is not provided, but the CDF of the MVN, F_ρ, is usually available. Hence, $F_\rho^{(k)}$ can be computed approximately using the numerical derivative

$$F_\rho^{(k)}(C_1, \ldots, C_K) \simeq \epsilon^{-1} \{ F_\rho(C_1, \ldots, C_k + \epsilon, \ldots, C_K) - F_\rho(C_1, \ldots, C_k, \ldots, C_K) \}$$

for a small ϵ. As a starting point, $C_K^{(0)}$, for the NR algorithm, it is convenient to use either (i) z_β, which has the same meaning as using n_0 in (4.4) or (ii) the solution of $G(C_K) = 0$ when $\gamma = (1, \ldots, 1)^T$. Many standard statistical software packages are already equipped with a macro to compute either (i) or (ii). In Appendices D.1 and D.2, respectively, we provide the codes for the R and SAS software packages needed to obtain C_K from this NR algorithm. Also, in order to find the solution C_K of the nonlinear equation (4.6), the R users can utilize the "optimize" function equipped in the R.

4.4 Numerical Tables for C_K

Consider the case of continuous endpoints (i.e., $a_1 = \cdots = a_K = 1$). In calculating the required sample size using the formula (4.5), where candidate values of δ_k's and ρ are available from pilot or historical data, the behaviour of $C_K = C_K(\beta, \rho, \gamma, \alpha)$ is complicated even if a computational algorithm for C_K is available. For investigators intending to use (4.5), it is convenient to have ready access to tables of values of C_K, which we provide for the frequently used cases of $K = 2$ and $K = 3$. The required sample size using (4.5) and tables of C_K can be computed even if a high computation environment is not available. To simplify these tables, without loss of generality, we assume that the rule

$$\gamma_1 \geq \gamma_2 \geq \cdots \geq \gamma_{K-1} \geq 1 \quad (\Leftrightarrow \quad \delta_1 \geq \delta_2 \geq \cdots \geq \delta_K)$$

is satisfied. Throughout this section, the significance level of $\alpha = 0.025$ is used.

4.4.1 Two Co-primary Endpoints

Using numerical tables for C_K provided by Tables 4.3 and 4.4 (see Sugimoto et al. 2012), we consider seven non-negative values of the correlation coefficient (ρ^{12}: 0, 0.2, 0.3, 0.5, 0.7, 0.8 and 0.95) and 15 effect size ratios (γ_1: 1.0, 1.02, 1.04, 1.07, 1.1, 1.13, 1.16, 1.2, 1.25, 1.3, 1.4, 1.5, 1.6, 1.8 and 2.0) when $\beta = 0.2$ and $\beta = 0.1$. The fine division for the effect size ratio is useful to improve the precision of linear interpolation for approximating the value of C_2 corresponding to γ_1 which does not fall under Tables 4.3 and 4.4.

Figure 4.2 shows the curves of $C_2(0.2, \rho^{12}, \gamma_1, 0.025)$ on ρ^{12} under the seven effect size ratios (γ_1: 1.0, 1.1, 1.2, 1.3, 1.4, 1.5 and 2.0). The curves of $C_2(0.1, \rho^{12}, \gamma_1, 0.025)$ tend to be similar to those in Fig. 4.2. Unless the correlation coefficient ρ^{12} is close to 1, using linear interpolation to approximate the missing C_2 values in Tables 4.3 and 4.4 is generally reasonable.

4.4.2 Three Co-primary Endpoints

When $\beta = 0.2$ and $\beta = 0.1$, using tables for C_K provided by Tables C.1 and C.2 in Appendix C (see Sugimoto et al. 2012), we consider 7 effect size ratios (γ_1, γ_2: 1.0, 1.1, 1.2, 1.3, 1.4, 1.5 and 2.0) and 4 levels of correlation, H(high, 0.8), M(medium, 0.5), L(low, 0.3) and 0 (none). However, because it would be excessive and not particularly useful to list all possible combinations of ρ^{12}, ρ^{13} and ρ^{23}, the table entries are restricted to the patterns with $\{\rho^{12} = \rho^{13} = \rho^{23}\}$, $\{0 < \rho^{12} = \rho^{13} \neq \rho^{23}\}$ and $\{\rho^{12} \neq \rho^{13} = \rho^{23} > 0\}$. The first pattern comprises H-H-H, M-M-M, L-L-L and 0-0-0 for the above patterns of correlation involving ρ^{12}-ρ^{13}-ρ^{23}. The second comprises H-H-M, H-H-L, M-M-H, M-M-L, L-L-H, L-L-M, M-M-0, L-L-0, and the third is in reverse order to the second; H-H-0 is excluded as an unrealized pattern because the determinant of the correlation matrix ρ with H-H-0 is negative. Tables C.1 and C.2 list the values of C_K calculated under these patterns (represented as H = 0.8, M = 0.5 and L = 0.3) of the correlation matrix

$$\rho = \begin{pmatrix} 1 & \rho^{12} & \rho^{13} \\ \rho^{12} & 1 & \rho^{23} \\ \rho^{13} & \rho^{23} & 1 \end{pmatrix}$$

and the two effect size ratios γ_1 ($= \delta_1/\delta_3$) and γ_2 ($= \delta_2/\delta_3$), when $\beta = 0.2$ and $\beta = 0.1$, respectively. In all combinations of ρ and $\gamma = (\gamma_1, \gamma_2)$ in Tables C.1 and C.2, the ratio of the required sample size at $\beta = 0.1$ to that at $\beta = 0.2$,

$$\frac{(C_3(0.1, \rho, \gamma, \alpha) + z_\alpha)^2}{(C_3(0.2, \rho, \gamma, \alpha) + z_\alpha)^2}|_{\alpha=0.025},$$

is between 1.22 and 1.34.

Table 4.3 $C_K(\beta, \rho^{12}, \gamma_1, \alpha)$ when $1 - \beta = 0.8$, $\alpha = 0.025$ and $K = 2$

γ_1	ρ^{12}						
	0.0	0.2	0.3	0.5	0.7	0.8	0.95
1.00	1.250	1.226	1.210	1.168	1.109	1.066	0.961
1.02	1.219	1.195	1.179	1.138	1.079	1.038	0.934
1.04	1.190	1.166	1.151	1.111	1.053	1.012	0.912
1.07	1.150	1.127	1.112	1.073	1.017	0.978	0.887
1.10	1.114	1.091	1.077	1.040	0.986	0.950	0.869
1.13	1.081	1.060	1.046	1.010	0.960	0.927	0.858
1.16	1.051	1.031	1.018	0.984	0.938	0.907	0.850
1.20	1.016	0.998	0.986	0.955	0.914	0.887	0.845
1.25	0.979	0.962	0.952	0.925	0.890	0.870	0.843
1.30	0.948	0.934	0.925	0.902	0.874	0.858	0.842
1.40	0.902	0.892	0.886	0.871	0.854	0.847	0.842
1.50	0.874	0.868	0.864	0.855	0.846	0.843	0.842
1.60	0.857	0.854	0.852	0.847	0.843	0.842	0.842
1.80	0.845	0.844	0.843	0.842	0.842	0.842	0.842
2.00	0.842	0.842	0.842	0.842	0.842	0.842	0.842

Table 4.4 $C_K(\beta, \rho^{12}, \gamma_1, \alpha)$ when $1 - \beta = 0.9$, $\alpha = 0.025$ and $K = 2$

γ_1	ρ^{12}						
	0.0	0.2	0.3	0.5	0.7	0.8	0.95
1.00	1.632	1.617	1.607	1.577	1.529	1.493	1.398
1.02	1.598	1.583	1.573	1.543	1.496	1.461	1.367
1.04	1.566	1.552	1.542	1.513	1.467	1.432	1.343
1.07	1.523	1.510	1.500	1.472	1.428	1.396	1.317
1.10	1.486	1.473	1.463	1.437	1.397	1.367	1.301
1.13	1.453	1.441	1.432	1.408	1.371	1.344	1.291
1.16	1.424	1.413	1.405	1.383	1.350	1.327	1.286
1.20	1.392	1.382	1.375	1.356	1.328	1.310	1.283
1.25	1.360	1.352	1.346	1.331	1.309	1.296	1.282
1.30	1.336	1.329	1.325	1.313	1.297	1.289	1.282
1.40	1.305	1.302	1.299	1.293	1.286	1.283	1.282
1.50	1.291	1.289	1.288	1.285	1.283	1.282	1.282
1.60	1.285	1.284	1.284	1.283	1.282	1.282	1.282
1.80	1.282	1.282	1.282	1.282	1.282	1.282	1.282
2.00	1.282	1.282	1.282	1.282	1.282	1.282	1.282

Fig. 4.2 The curves of $C_2(0.2, \rho^{12}, \gamma_1, 0.025)$ on ρ^{12} under $\gamma_1 = 1.0, 1.1, 1.2, 1.3, 1.4, 1.5, 2.0$

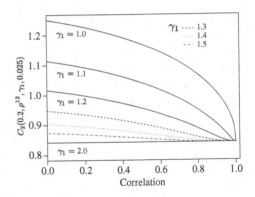

4.4.3 Computational Note

To create the tables for C_K in Sugimoto et al. (2012), the CDF of the K-variate MVN is computed using the method developed by Miwa et al. (2003), where the number of grid points is set to 512 to better approximate the value of the CDF. Furthermore, it is confirmed that the C_K values are the same as the simulated averages obtained from using the method by Genz (1992) with $\varepsilon = 10^{-6}$, where ε is an absolute error tolerance to stop the repetition in his method based on a Monte-Carlo procedure.

4.5 Examples

As discussed in Sect. 2.6 and the related guideline (CHMP 2008), a typical clinical trial for Alzheimer's disease (AD) is a randomized, double-blind, placebo-controlled, parallel group clinical trial with cognitive, functional and global endpoints to evaluate a symptomatic improvement in the dementia caused by the disease. These endpoints may be classified as follows:

(i) objective cognitive tests, e.g. ADAS-cog (AD Assessment Scale cognitive sub-scale) and SIB (Severe Impairment Battery);

(ii) self-care and activities of daily living, e.g. ADCS-ADL (AD Cooperative Study Activities of Daily Living) and its modified version for severe AD; and

(iii) global assessment of change, such as CIBIC-plus (Clinician's Interview Based Impression of Change-plus) and CGI-I (Clinical Global Impression of Improvement).

For illustration, we first consider the case of two co-primary endpoints and then consider a case of three co-primary endpoints. The data used for calculation are taken from Rogers et al. (1998) and Winblad et al. (2006).

4.5.1 Two Co-primary Endpoints

For the case of two co-primary endpoints, we refer to the results obtained by Rogers et al. (1998). Based on the results, the standardized effect sizes of the changes in ADAS-cog score from the baseline and the CIBIC-plus at the final visit are estimated to be 0.47 and 0.48, respectively. Thus, in designing a future study to compare two treatments (Donepezil vs. Placebo), we consider the case of $\delta_1 = 0.48$ and $\delta_2 = 0.47$ (according the rule of $\delta_1 \geq \delta_2$) with $\rho^{12} = 0, 0.3, 0.5, 0.8$, $\alpha = 0.025$ and $\beta = 0.2$. Given that $\gamma_1 = \delta_1/\delta_2 \simeq 1.021$, we use $C_2 = 1.219, 1.179, 1.138, 1.038$ from Table 4.3 for each value of ρ^{12}. Hence, the equal sample sizes per group $n = n_T = n_C$ (i.e., $r = 1.0$) were calculated from (4.5) as follows:

$$
n = \begin{cases}
2(1.219 + 1.96)^2/0.47^2 = 91.50 \rightarrow 92 \text{ if } \rho^{12} = 0.0 \\
2(1.179 + 1.96)^2/0.47^2 = 89.21 \rightarrow 90 \text{ if } \rho^{12} = 0.3 \\
2(1.138 + 1.96)^2/0.47^2 = 86.90 \rightarrow 87 \text{ if } \rho^{12} = 0.5 \\
2(1.038 + 1.96)^2/0.47^2 = 81.38 \rightarrow 82 \text{ if } \rho^{12} = 0.8
\end{cases}
$$

As a second example, consider the study of Winblad et al. (2006) to compare two treatments (Donepezil vs. Placebo). The two co-primary endpoints are the changes from the baseline to month six in the SIB score and ADCS-ADL-severe (a modified ADCS-ADL for severe AD). They calculated the required sample size per group as follows:

... we needed a sample size of 101 patients per treatment group to detect with 90 % power an absolute difference between treatments in ADCS-ADL-severe of 3.5 (SD = 7.6) with α level of 0.05. With the same power and significance level, we needed to enroll 86 patients per group to detect a 7 (SD = 14) point absolute treatment difference in SIB scores ...

This means that, by randomizing 101 patients per group to test (4.1) with $\alpha = 0.025$, the statistical power of at least $0.9 \times 0.9 = 0.81$ (more precisely, $0.9 \times 0.94 = 0.846$) is assured even if the SIB score and ADCS-ADL-severe are uncorrelated. Now, we use Tables 4.3 and 4.4 for the effect sizes of $\delta_1 = 0.5$ (SIB) and $\delta_2 = 0.46$ (ADCS-ADL-severe). Given that $\gamma_1 = \delta_1/\delta_2 \simeq 1.087$, we use linear interpolation between the values of C_2 at $\gamma_1 = 1.07$ and 1.10 from Tables 4.3 and 4.4. When $\alpha = 0.025$, the equal sample sizes per group $n = n_T = n_C$ (i.e., $r = 1.0$) calculated from (4.5) are

$$
n = \begin{cases}
2\left(\frac{0.013}{0.030}1.150 + \frac{0.017}{0.030}1.114 + 1.96\right)^2/0.46^2 \rightarrow 91 \text{ if } \rho^{12} = 0.0, \ \beta = 0.2 \\
2\left(\frac{0.013}{0.030}1.073 + \frac{0.017}{0.030}1.040 + 1.96\right)^2/0.46^2 \rightarrow 86 \text{ if } \rho^{12} = 0.5, \ \beta = 0.2 \\
2\left(\frac{0.013}{0.030}1.523 + \frac{0.017}{0.030}1.486 + 1.96\right)^2/0.46^2 \rightarrow 114 \text{ if } \rho^{12} = 0.0, \ \beta = 0.1 \\
2\left(\frac{0.013}{0.030}1.472 + \frac{0.017}{0.030}1.437 + 1.96\right)^2/0.46^2 \rightarrow 111 \text{ if } \rho^{12} = 0.5, \ \beta = 0.1
\end{cases}
$$

which are identical to the numbers computed exactly for $\gamma_1 = 1.087$ using the NR algorithm described in Sect. 4.3.

4.5.2 Three Co-primary Endpoints

For illustration, consider a clinical trial for AD with the three co-primary endpoints, the SIB score (an objective cognitive test), ADCS-ADL-severe (self-care and activities of daily living) and the CGI-I score for global assessment of change.

From the results of a modified intention-to-treat population, the estimated standardized effect sizes of the changes from the baseline to month six in SIB score, ADCS-ADL-severe and CGI-I score are 0.36, 0.30 and 0.26, respectively. Based on these values, consider the case of $\delta = (0.36, 0.30, 0.26)^T$ with $\rho = \rho_M, \rho_L, \rho_N$, $\alpha = 0.025$ and $\beta = 0.2$, where

$$\rho_v = \begin{pmatrix} 1 & v & v \\ v & 1 & v \\ v & v & 1 \end{pmatrix}, \quad v : M = 0.5, \ L = 0.3, \ N = 0.0.$$

Given $\gamma_1 = 1.385$ and $\gamma_2 = 1.154$, for values of C_3 at $\gamma = (1.3, 1.1)$ and $(1.4, 1.2)$ in Table C.1, we approximate the values of $C_3^{(1.385, 1.154)}$ using the linear interpolation

$$\frac{0.046}{0.100} \left\{ \frac{0.015}{0.100} C_3^{(1.3,1.1)} + \frac{0.085}{0.100} C_3^{(1.4,1.1)} \right\} + \frac{0.054}{0.100} \left\{ \frac{0.015}{0.100} C_3^{(1.3,1.2)} + \frac{0.085}{0.100} C_3^{(1.4,1.2)} \right\},$$

where $C_3^{(\gamma_1, \gamma_2)}$ is an abbreviation of $C_3(\beta, \rho, \gamma, \alpha)$. For example, if $\rho = \rho_M$, $C_3^{(1.3,1.1)}$, $C_3^{(1.4,1.1)}$, $C_3^{(1.3,1.2)}$ and $C_3^{(1.4,1.2)}$ are, from Table C.1, 1.065, 1.050, 0.990 and 0.970, respectively. Hence, from (4.5), the required sample sizes per group are approximately

$$n = \begin{cases} 2(1.009 + 1.96)^2/0.26^2 = 260.8 \to 261 & \text{if} \quad \rho = \rho_M \\ 2(1.050 + 1.96)^2/0.26^2 = 268.1 \to 269 & \text{if} \quad \rho = \rho_L \\ 2(1.091 + 1.96)^2/0.26^2 = 275.4 \to 276 & \text{if} \quad \rho = \rho_N \end{cases},$$

which exceed the numbers of patients computed exactly for $\gamma = (1.385, 1.154)$ by only one. The exact values of $C_3^{(1.385, 1.154)}$ are 1.004, 1.045 and 1.086 at $\rho = \rho_M$, ρ_L and ρ_N, respectively. The linear interpolation gives a conservative approximation for the sample size in general because C_K is convex on $\{\gamma : \gamma_1, \dots, \gamma_{K-1} \geq 1\}$.

In all cases of $K \geq 4$, and in other cases of $K = 2$ or $K = 3$ in which ρ and γ are not compatible with the conditions implied by Tables 4.3 to C.2, investigators can compute C_K, the solution of (4.6), using the codes for the R and SAS software packages provided in Appendices D.1 and D.2.

4.6 Summary

This chapter provides convenient formulae and numerical tables for sample size calculations associated with designing clinical trials with two interventions when all of the endpoints are either continuous or binary. The formulae and numerical tables provide a practical tool for implementing the methods discussed in Chaps. 2 and 3. The major points are as follows:

- The formulae are natural extensions to existing formulae for the univariate case in both the continuous and binary endpoint cases. The methods are easy to implement in practice using the numerical tables or an algorithm for C_K.
- The formulae provide a clear picture of the relationship between the factors (e.g., type I and II errors, effect sizes, correlations and variances) and reveal how the sample size is influenced by these factors.
- An NR algorithm is provided for obtaining C_K for arbitrary values of the type I and II errors, effect size ratios, and correlations. The NR algorithm usually completes the calculation with a smaller number of steps than the procedure in which the tentative sample size is consecutively updated until achieving the target power. Using the algorithm, in all cases of $K \geq 4$, and in other cases of $K = 2$ or $K = 3$ in which the correlations and the effect size ratios are not compatible with the conditions presented in the prepared tables, investigators can compute C_K using the R and SAS codes provided in Appendices D.1 and D.2.

References

Bartlett MS (1947) The use of transformations. Biometrics 3:39–52

Committee for Medicinal Products for Human Use (CHMP) (2008) Guideline on medicinal products for the treatment Alzheimer's disease and other dementias (CPMP/EWP/553/95 Rev.1). EMEA: London. http://www.ema.europa.eu/docs/en_GB/document_library/Scientific_guideline/2009/09/WC500003562.pdf. Accessed 9 June 2014

Genz A (1992) Numerical computation of multivariate normal probabilities. J Comput Graph Stat 1:141–150

Miwa A, Hayter J, Kuriki S (2003) The evaluation of general non-centred orthant probabilities. J R Stat Soc B 65:223–234

Pearson K (1900) On the criterion that a given system of deviations from the probable in the case of a correlated system of variables is such that it can be reasonably supposed to have arisen from random sampling. Philos Mag, Ser B 50:157–175

Rogers SL, Farlow MR, Doody RS, Mohs R, Friedhoff LT (1998) The donepezil study group. A 24-week, double-blind, placebo-controlled trial of donepezil in patients with Alzheimer's disease. Neurology 50:136–145

Sozu T, Sugimoto T, Hamasaki T (2010) Sample size determination in clinical trials with multiple co-primary binary endpoints. Stat Med 29:2169–2179

Sozu T, Sugimoto T, Hamasaki T (2011) Sample size determination in superiority clinical trials with multiple co-primary correlated endpoints. J Biopharm Stat 21:650–668

Sugimoto T, Sozu T, Hamasaki T (2012) A convenient formula for sample size calculations in clinical trials with multiple co-primary continuous endpoints. Biopharm Stat 11:118–128

Walters DE (1979) In defence of the arc sine approximation. Stat 28:219–222

Winblad B, Kilander L, Eriksson S, Minthon L, Batsman S, Wetterholmf AL, Jansson-Blixt C, Haglund A (2006) Donepezil in patients with severe Alzheimer's disease: double-blind, parallel-group, placebo-controlled study. Lancet 367:1057–1065

Yates F (1934) Contingency tables involving small numbers and the χ^2 test. J R Stat Soc, Suppl 1:217–235

Chapter 5
Continuous Primary Endpoints

Abstract In this chapter, we provide an overview of the concepts and technical fundamentals regarding power and sample size calculation for clinical trials comparing two interventions with multiple continuous outcomes as multiple primary endpoints. There are many procedures for controlling the type I error rate. We discuss the simplest procedure, the unstructured Bonferroni procedure as it is well-known and widely utilized in practice. We evaluate the behavior of the sample size and power associated with the methods. We introduce conservative sample sizing strategies in these clinical trials and provide numerical examples for illustration.

Keywords Bonferroni procedure · Conservative sample size · Disjunctive power · Multivariate normal · Union intersection test

5.1 Introduction

In this chapter, we discuss a situation in which the sample size is selected based on an alternative hypothesis that an effect exists for AT LEAST ONE endpoint. There are many procedures for controlling type I error rate. We will discuss the simplest procedure, the unstructured Bonferroni procedure as it is well-known and widely used in practice.

Consider a randomized clinical trial comparing two interventions with n_T subjects in the test group and n_C subjects in the control group. There are $K (\geq 2)$ continuous endpoints with a K-variate normal distribution. There is interest in evaluating an alternative hypothesis of superiority for AT LEAST ONE of the endpoints. The type I error rate needs to be controlled adequately since the type I error rate increases as the number of endpoints to be evaluated increases. One of the methods for controlling the type I error rate is the Bonferroni procedure, a well-known and simple procedure that is frequently used in practice. The Bonferroni procedure equally distributes the type I error rate α among the endpoints. For example with K continuous endpoints, each endpoint would be tested at $\alpha_k = \alpha/K$ $(k = 1, \ldots, K)$. We are now interested in testing $H_0 : \delta_k \leq 0$ for all k versus $H_1 : \delta_k > 0$ for at least one k at the (overall) significance level of α, based on the test statistics $(Z_1, \ldots, Z_K)^T$, the same

© The Author(s) 2015

T. Sozu et al., *Sample Size Determination in Clinical Trials with Multiple Endpoints*, SpringerBriefs in Statistics, DOI 10.1007/978-3-319-22005-5_5

statistics defined in Sect. 2.2.1. However, the rejection regions of H_0 are $[\{Z_1 > z_{\alpha/K}\} \cup \cdots \cup \{Z_K > z_{\alpha/K}\}]$ if the variances are assumed to be known. However, the Bonferroni procedure is conservative especially when there are many highly correlated endpoints to be evaluated (Dmitrienko et al. 2010; Senn and Bretz 2007).

For the standardized effect size δ_k, the overall power is

$$1 - \beta = \Pr\left[\bigcup_{k=1}^{K}\{Z_k > z_{\alpha/K}\} \,\middle|\, H_1\right] = 1 - \Pr\left[\bigcap_{k=1}^{K}\{Z_k \le z_{\alpha/K}\} \,\middle|\, H_1\right]$$

$$= 1 - \Pr\left[\bigcap_{k=1}^{K}\{Z_k^* \le c_k^*\} \,\middle|\, H_1\right] \tag{5.1}$$

where Z_k^* are the same statistics as defined in Sect. 2.2.1 and $c_k^* = z_{\alpha/K} - \sqrt{\kappa n}\delta_k$. This overall power (5.1) is referred to as "minimal power" (Westfall et al. 2011) or "disjunctive power" (Bretz et al. 2011; Senn and Bretz 2007). The overall power (5.1) is calculated by using the cumulative distribution function of the K-variate normal distribution with zero mean vector and correlation matrix ρ_Z with off-diagonal elements given by $\rho^{kk'}$ as in Sect. 2.2.1. The sample size required to achieve the desired overall power of $1 - \beta$ at the significance level of α is the smallest integer not less than n satisfying (5.1).

5.2 Behavior of the Type I Error Rate, Power and Sample Size

We focus on the behavior of the type I error rate, overall power and sample size calculated when designing a trial with an alternative hypothesis of superiority for AT LEAST ONE endpoint.

5.2.1 Type I Error Rate

It is known that the type I error rate is below the nominal error rate when the endpoints are positively and highly correlated (Dmitrienko et al. 2010). Figure 5.1 illustrates the behavior of type I error rate as a function of the correlation, where the off-diagonal elements of the correlation matrix are equal, i.e., $\rho = \rho^{12} = \cdots = \rho^{K-1,K}$, all of the standardized effect sizes are zero, i.e., $\delta_1 = \cdots = \delta_K = 0$ ($K = 2, 3, 4, 5,$ and 10), and the Bonferroni adjustment is applied at the significance level of $\alpha = 0.025$. This behavior is discussed in Dmitrienko et al. (2010). Given this result, an adjustment to sample size may be considered when a high positive correlation is expected.

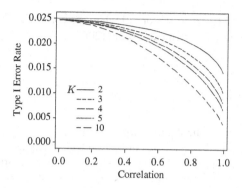

Fig. 5.1 Behavior of the type I error rate as a function of the correlation, where the off-diagonal elements of the correlation matrix are equal, i.e., $\rho = \rho^{12} = \cdots = \rho^{K-1,K}$ and all of the standardized effect sizes are zero, i.e., $\delta_1 = \cdots = \delta_K = 0$. The Bonferroni adjustment is applied at the significance level of $\alpha = 0.025$

5.2.2 Overall Power

Figure 5.2 illustrates how the overall power behaves as a function of correlation for a given sample size, where the off-diagonal elements of the correlation matrix are equal, i.e., $\rho = \rho^{12} = \cdots = \rho^{K-1,K}$, and all of the standardized effect sizes are equal to 0.2, i.e., $\delta_1 = \cdots = \delta_K = 0.2$. In addition, the Bonferroni adjustment is applied and the power for each one-sided adjusted individual test at a significance level of $\alpha = 0.025$ is 0.80 and 0.90. The figure illustrates that the power increases with more endpoints if the correlation is less than $\rho = 0.7$, while the power is less

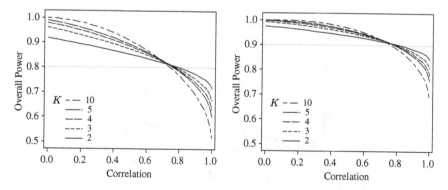

Fig. 5.2 Behavior of the overall power $1 - \beta$ as a function of the correlation for a given sample size, where the off-diagonal elements of the correlation matrix are equal, i.e., $\rho = \rho^{12} = \cdots = \rho^{K-1,K}$, and all of the standardized effect sizes are equal to 0.2, i.e., $\delta_1 = \cdots = \delta_K = 0.2$. The Bonferroni adjustment is applied and the power for each one-sided adjusted individual test at a significance level of $\alpha = 0.025$ is 0.80 and 0.90

than desired power of $1 - \beta = 0.8$ or 0.9 when the correlation is greater than 0.7. This behavior is discussed in Senn and Bretz (2007).

5.2.3 Sample Size

Figure 5.3 illustrates how the equal sample size per group $n(\rho) = n_T = n_C$ (i.e., $r = 1.0$) behaves as a function of the correlation when there are K endpoints ($K = 2, 3, 4, 5$, and 10), where the off-diagonal elements of the correlation matrix are equal $\rho = \rho^{12} = \cdots = \rho^{K-1,K}$, all of the standardized effect sizes are equal to 0.2, i.e., $\delta_1 = \cdots = \delta_K = 0.2$ was calculated with the overall power of $1 - \beta = 0.80$ when each of the K endpoints is tested at the significance level of $\alpha = 0.025/K$ by a one-sided test with Bonferroni adjustment. The vertical axis is the ratio of $n(\rho)$ to $n(0)$. The figure illustrates that the ratio becomes lager as the correlation approaches one and the degree of increase is larger as the number of endpoints to be evaluated increases.

Figure 5.4 illustrates how the equal sample size per group $n = n_T = n_C$ (i.e., $r = 1.0$) behaves as a function of the correlation when there are two endpoints ($K = 2$), where $\delta_2/\delta_1 = 1.0, 1.25, 1.50, 1.75$, and 2.0; when each of two endpoints is tested at the significance level of $\alpha = 0.025/2$ by a one-sided test with Bonferroni adjustment. The vertical axis is the ratio of $n(\rho^{12})$ to $n(0)$. When $\delta_2/\delta_1 = 1.0$, the ratio of the required sample size increases as the correlation approaches one, as seen in Fig. 5.3. Even when $1.0 < \delta_2/\delta_1 < 1.5$, the ratio of the required sample size still increases as the correlation approaches one. However, when the ratio δ_2/δ_1 exceeds 1.5, the sample size does not change considerably as the correlation varies.

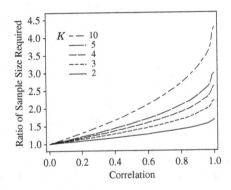

Fig. 5.3 Behavior of the sample size $n(\rho)$ as a function of the correlation for a given sample size, where the off-diagonal elements of the correlation matrix are equal $\rho = \rho^{12} = \cdots = \rho^{K-1,K}$, and all of the standardized effect sizes are equal to 0.2, i.e., $\delta_1 = \cdots = \delta_K = 0.2$ ($K = 2, 3, 4, 5$, and 10). The sample size was calculated to evaluate an alternative hypothesis of superiority for AT LEAST ONE endpoint with the overall power of $1 - \beta = 0.80$ for a one-sided test at the significance level of $\alpha = 0.025/K$, where the Bonferroni adjustment was applied

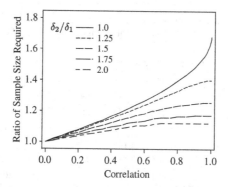

Fig. 5.4 Behavior of the required sample size as a function of the correlation $n(\rho^{12})$ when there are two endpoints as primary. The *vertical* axis is the ratio of $n(\rho^{12})$ to $n(0)$. The equal sample sizes per group $n = n_T = n_C$ (i.e., $r = 1.0$) were calculated to detect superiority for at least one endpoint, with the overall power of $1 - \beta = 0.80$ at the significance level of $\alpha = 0.025/2$, where the Bonferroni adjustment was applied

Table 5.1 provides the required sample sizes for trials with two primary endpoints with correlation $\rho^{12} = 0.0$ (no correlation), 0.3 (low correlation), 0.5 (moderate correlation), and 0.8 (high correlation), where the equal sample sizes $n = n_T = n_C$ (i.e., $r = 1.0$) were calculated to detect standardized effect sizes of $0.2 \leq \delta_1, \delta_2 \leq 0.4$ with the overall power of $1 - \beta = 0.80$ and 0.90, when each of the two endpoints is tested at the significance level of $\alpha = 0.025/2$ by a one-sided test. As seen in Fig. 5.4, when the effect sizes for the two endpoints are equal, the required sample size increases as the correlation approaches one. Comparing the cases of $\rho^{12} = 0.0$ and $\rho^{12} = 0.8$, the increase in the sample size is approximately 40 % in both of the $1 - \beta = 0.80$ and 0.90 cases. Even in the cases of unequal effect sizes, that is $\delta_1 < \delta_2$, the sample sizes increases as the correlation approaches one. However, when the ratio δ_2/δ_1 exceeds roughly 1.5, the required sample size does not change considerably as a function of the correlation. When $\delta_2/\delta_1 = 1.5$, the increase in the sample size is approximately 24 % in both of the $1 - \beta = 0.80$ and 0.90, and 12 % when $\delta_2/\delta_1 = 2.0$.

Similar to the case of two endpoints, Table 5.2 provides the required sample size for three primary endpoints ($K = 3$), where the equal sample sizes per group $n = n_T = n_C$ (i.e., $r = 1.0$) were calculated to detect standardized effect sizes of $0.2 \leq \delta_1, \delta_2, \delta_3 \leq 0.4$ with the overall power of $1 - \beta = 0.80$ and 0.90, when each of the three endpoints is tested at the significance level of $\alpha = 0.025/3$ by a one-sided test, and the off-diagonal elements of the correlation matrix are equal, i.e., $\rho = \rho^{12} = \rho^{13} = \rho^{23} = 0.0, 0.3, 0.5,$ and 0.8. Similarly as seen in Table 5.1, when the effect sizes of the three endpoints are equal, the required sample size increases as the correlation approaches one. Comparing the cases of $\rho = 0.0$ and $\rho = 0.8$, the increase in the sample size is approximately 67 % when $1 - \beta = 0.80$ and 70 % when $1 - \beta = 0.90$. Even when effect sizes are unequal, that is $\delta_1 < \delta_2 \leq \delta_3$, the sample size still increases as the correlation approaches one. However, when the ratios δ_2/δ_1

Table 5.1 The required equal sample sizes per group $n = n_T = n_C$ (i.e., $r = 1.0$) for two endpoints with the overall power of $1 - \beta = 0.80$ and 0.9 at the significance level of $\alpha = 0.025/2$, where the Bonferroni adjustment was applied

Targeted power	Standardized effect size		Correlation ρ^{12}					E_1	E_2
	δ_1	δ_2	0.0	0.3	0.5	0.8	1.0		
0.80	0.20	0.20	282	316	342	394	476	476	476
	0.20	0.25	218	243	260	290	305	476	305
	0.20	0.30	169	185	195	209	212	476	212
	0.20	0.35	133	143	149	155	156	476	156
	0.20	0.40	106	112	116	119	119	476	119
	0.25	0.25	181	203	219	252	305	305	305
	0.25	0.30	147	164	177	199	212	305	212
	0.25	0.35	120	132	140	152	156	305	156
	0.25	0.40	98	107	112	118	119	305	119
	0.30	0.30	126	141	152	175	212	212	212
	0.30	0.35	106	118	128	144	156	212	156
	0.30	0.40	89	99	105	116	119	212	119
	0.35	0.35	93	104	112	129	156	156	156
	0.35	0.40	89	99	105	116	119	156	119
	0.40	0.40	71	79	86	99	119	119	119
0.90	0.20	0.20	370	419	455	522	621	621	621
	0.20	0.25	287	321	345	383	398	621	398
	0.20	0.30	222	244	258	274	276	621	276
	0.20	0.35	174	188	196	203	203	621	203
	0.20	0.40	139	148	152	156	156	621	156
	0.25	0.25	237	268	291	334	398	398	398
	0.25	0.30	193	217	234	262	276	398	276
	0.25	0.35	157	174	185	200	203	398	203
	0.25	0.40	129	141	148	155	156	398	156
	0.30	0.30	165	186	202	232	276	276	276
	0.30	0.35	139	156	169	191	203	276	203
	0.30	0.40	117	130	139	152	156	276	156
	0.35	0.35	121	137	149	171	203	203	203
	0.35	0.40	117	130	139	152	156	203	156
	0.40	0.40	93	105	114	131	156	156	156

E_1, E_2: Sample size separately calculated for each endpoint 1 and 2 so that the individual power is at least 0.8 and 0.9 at $\alpha = 0.025/2$

and δ_3/δ_1 exceed 1.5, the required sample size does not change as the correlation varies. When $\delta_2/\delta_1 = \delta_3/\delta_1 = 1.5$, the increase in the sample size is approximately 53 % when $1 - \beta = 0.80$ and 52 % when $1 - \beta = 0.90$. When $\delta_2/\delta_1 = \delta_3/\delta_1 = 2.0$, it is approximately 44 % when $1 - \beta = 0.80$ and 41 % when $1 - \beta = 0.90$.

Table 5.2 The required sample size per group ($n = n_T = n_C$, $r = 1.0$) for three endpoints with the overall power of $1 - \beta = 0.80$ and 0.9 at $\alpha = 0.025$, assuming that the variance is known

Targeted power	Standarized effect size			Correlation ρ^{12}							
	δ_1	δ_2	δ_3	0.0	0.3	0.5	0.8	1.0	E_1	E_2	E_3
0.80	0.20	0.20	0.20	238	285	323	398	524	524	524	524
	0.20	0.20	0.30	162	188	206	230	233	524	524	233
	0.20	0.20	0.40	108	120	126	131	131	524	524	131
	0.20	0.30	0.30	127	149	166	194	233	524	233	233
	0.20	0.30	0.40	93	107	116	128	131	524	233	131
	0.20	0.40	0.40	76	87	95	110	131	524	131	131
	0.30	0.30	0.30	106	127	144	177	233	233	233	233
	0.30	0.30	0.40	83	98	108	126	131	233	233	131
	0.30	0.40	0.40	69	82	91	109	131	233	131	131
	0.40	0.40	0.40	60	72	81	100	131	131	131	131
0.90	0.20	0.20	0.20	309	376	427	525	676	676	676	676
	0.20	0.20	0.30	211	247	270	298	301	676	676	301
	0.20	0.20	0.40	140	156	164	169	169	676	676	169
	0.20	0.30	0.30	165	196	218	254	301	676	301	301
	0.20	0.30	0.40	121	140	152	166	169	676	301	169
	0.20	0.40	0.40	98	114	125	143	169	676	131	169
	0.30	0.30	0.30	138	168	190	234	301	301	301	301
	0.30	0.30	0.40	107	128	143	164	169	301	301	169
	0.30	0.40	0.40	90	108	121	143	169	301	131	169
	0.40	0.40	0.40	78	94	107	132	169	131	131	169

E_1, E_2, E_3: Sample size separately calculated for each endpoint 1, 2, and 3 so that the individual power is at least 0.8 and 0.9 at $\alpha = 0.025/3$

5.3 Conservative Sample Size Determination

Similarly, as in the previous section, consider a conservative sample size determination for evaluating an alternative hypothesis of superiority for AT LEAST ONE endpoint when there are two primary endpoints. As the overall power is lowest when $\rho^{12} = 1$, we may set

$$1 - \beta = \Phi_2(-c_1^*, \infty \mid \rho^{12} = 1) + \Phi_2(\infty, -c_2^* \mid \rho^{12} = 1) - \Phi_2(-c_1^*, -c_2^* \mid \rho^{12} = 1), \quad (5.2)$$

where $\Phi_2(\cdot)$ is cumulative distribution function of a bivariate normal distribution with zero mean and correlation matrix with off-diagonal element ρ^{12}. Using the result in

Owen (1962, 1965), we can rewrite the overall power (5.2) using the univariate standard normal distribution function. It is given by

$$1 - \beta = \begin{cases} \Phi(-c_1^*), & c_1^* > c_2^*, \\ \Phi(-c_2^*), & c_1^* \leq c_2^*. \end{cases}$$

If we assume a un-pooled variance under the alternative hypothesis, then this leads to the conservative value of n given by

$$n_{CNSV} = \min \left\{ \frac{(z_{\alpha/2} + z_\beta)^2}{\kappa \delta_1^2}, \frac{(z_{\alpha/2} + z_\beta)^2}{\kappa \delta_2^2} \right\}$$

The sample size n_{CNSV} may be unnecessarily conservative as the assumption of $\rho^{12} = 1$ is often unrealistic in practice. Alternatively, we may consider the sample size $n_{CNSV}(\rho^{12})$ with $\rho^* < \rho^{12} < 1$, where ρ^* is a boundary value of the correlation in which a power is less than desired power.

5.4 Example

We illustrate the sample size calculations when the alternative hypothesis is superiority for at least one endpoint. Consider the clinical trial for the treatment of Alzheimer's disease from Rogers et al. (1998), discussed in Sect. 2.6. The study is a 24-week, double-blind, placebo-controlled trial of donepezil in patients with Alzheimer's disease and the primary efficacy endpoints were the cognitive portion of the Alzheimer's Disease Assessment Scale (ADAS-cog) and the Clinician's Interview Based Assessment of Change-Plus (CIBIC plus). From the result in Rogers et al. (1998), the absolute values of the standardized effect size with 95 % confidence interval were estimated as 0.47 (0.24, 0.69) for ADAS-cog (Endpoint 1: δ_1) and 0.48 (0.25, 0.70) for CIBIC-plus (Endpoint 2: δ_2). On the basis of these estimates, the sample size was calculated to detect the standardized effect sizes $0.20 < \delta_1, \delta_2 < 0.70$ to achieve the overall power of $1 - \beta = 0.80$ at $\alpha = 0.025$ with $\rho^{12} = 0.0, 0.3, 0.8$ and 1.0 as the correlation between ADAS-cog and CIBIC-plus. Figure 5.5 displays contour plots of the required sample sizes per group with two effect sizes δ_1 and δ_2 and correlation ρ^{12}. As the baseline case of $(\delta_1, \delta_2) = (0.47, 0.48)$, the sample sizes per group for $\rho^{12} = 0, 0.3, 0.8$ and 1.0 were 50, 56, 70, and 83, respectively. In this situation, as a conservative option, assuming a correlation of 1.0 between the two endpoints, a size of 83 is recommended and it is 1.66 times larger than that given by assuming zero correlation.

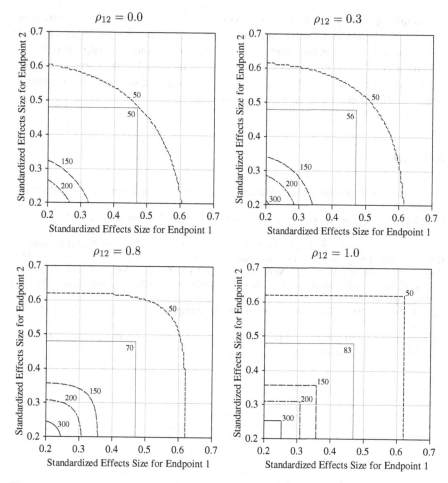

Fig. 5.5 Contour plots of sample size (per group) for standardized effect sizes of endpoint 1 (SIB-J) and endpoint 2 (CIBIC plus-J) with $\rho^{12} = 0.0, 0.3, 0.8$ and 1.0. The sample size was calculated to evaluate the alternative hypothesis of superiority for at least one endpoint with the overall power of $1 - \beta = 0.80$ for a one-sided test at the significance level of $\alpha = 0.025/2$ where the Bonferroni adjustment was applied

5.5 Summary

This chapter provides an overview of concepts and technical fundamentals regarding power and sample size determination for clinical trials with multiple continuous endpoints designed to evaluate superiority for AT LEAST ONE continuous endpoint with the simplest procedure, i.e., the unstructured Bonferroni procedure.

The behaviors of power and sample size for evaluating superiority for at least one endpoint with unstructured Bonferroni procedure are very different from those for evaluating superiority for all endpoints. As seen in Fig. 5.2, the power is improved as the number of endpoints to be evaluated is increased as the correlation goes toward zero from about 0.7. On the other hand, when the endpoints are highly correlated, the power is worse as the number of endpoints is increased as the correlation goes toward one from about 0.7. As seen in Fig. 5.3, the required sample size is increased as the number of endpoints is increased and as the correlation goes toward one.

References

Bretz F, Hothorn T, Westfall P (2011) Multiple comparisons using. Chapman & Hall/CRC, Boca Raton

Dmitrienko A, Tamhane AC, Bretz F (2010) Multiple testing problems in pharmaceutical statistics. Chapman & Hall/CRC, Boca Raton

Owen DB (1962) Handbook of statistical tables. Reading: Addison-Wesley Publishing Company

Owen DB (1965) A special case of the bivariate non-central t-distribution. Biometrika 52:437–446

Rogers SL, Farlow MR, Doody RS, Mohs R, Friedhoff LT (1998) The Donepezil Study Group. A 24-week, double-blind, placebo-controlled trial of donepezil in patients with Alzheimer's disease. Neurology 50:136–145

Senn S, Bretz F (2007) Power and sample size when multiple endpoints are considered. Pharma Stat 6:161–170

Westfall PH, Tobias RD, Wolfinger RD (2011) Multiple comparisons and multiple tests using SAS, 2nd edn. Cary: SAS Institute Inc

Chapter 6
Further Developments

Abstract In this book, we have focused our discussion on methods for sample size calculation in clinical trials with co-primary endpoints, although we have briefly discussed methods for clinical trials with multiple endpoints using the Bonferroni procedure. These discussions have been based on trials with superiority hypotheses, two intervention groups, no formal interim analyses, and continuous or binary endpoints. In this chapter, we briefly discuss developments for designing randomized trials with other design characteristics including: (i) other inferential goals, (ii) more than two intervention groups, (iii) group sequential designs, and (iv) endpoints with other measurement scales such as time to-event.

Keywords Global procedure · Group-sequential designs · Multiple-arm · Time-to-event · Superiority-noninferiority procedures

This book discusses methods for power and sample size determination for comparing the effect of two interventions in superiority clinical trials with multiple endpoints. The discussion focuses on methods for sample size calculation in clinical trials when the aim is to evaluate effects on ALL endpoints although we briefly discuss methods to evaluate effects on AT LEAST ONE endpoint using the Bonferroni procedure.

Clinical trial endpoints can exhibit several scales of measurement including continuous, binary, ordinal, and event-time. In this book, we discuss methods for addressing situations where: (1) all of the endpoints are continuous, and (2) all of the endpoints are binary. However the methods described in this book provide the foundation for designing randomized trials with other design characteristics, including clinical trials with (i) other inferential goals, (ii) more than two intervention groups, (iii) group sequential designs, and (iv) other endpoint measurement scales such as time-to-event. In addition, there may be instances where the co-primary endpoints are of mixed scales of measurement. For example, a trial evaluating interventions for pain may have pain evaluated on a continuous scale (e.g., Gracely pain scale) but have a binary safety endpoint (occurance of an adverse event). We briefly discuss these scenarios.

Other Inferential Goals

Dmitrienko et al. (2010) define the four types of inferential goals for analysis of multiple endpoints in clinical trials, i.e., all-or-none, at-least-one, global, and superiority-noninferiority procedures. This book discusses methods for the first two goals. The global procedure evaluates if the test intervention has an overall effect across the endpoints compared with the control intervention, but does not necessarily evaluate the effect on any specific endpoint. The procedure is conceptually similar to composite endpoints (Dmitrienko et al. 2010). The sample size may be calculated based on the T^2-test statistics. The goal of the superiority-noninferiority procedure is to evaluate if the test intervention is superior to the control intervention on at least one endpoint, but not inferior on all other endpoints (Bloch et al. 2001; Röhmel et al. 2006). This is an important goal when evaluating interventions for diseases with existing interventions but the interventions have only modest efficacy, concerning toxicity, or are very costly. The sample size methods discussed in this book are useful when considering sample size methods in the superiority-noninferiority procedure.

More Than Two Interventions

Designs with more than two interventions are common in many applications such as dose response trials. The methods discussed in this book can be conceptually generalized to such clinical trials, but the situation is complicated by the need for prespecified incorporation of multiple testing strategies.

Group Sequential Designs

In most conventional clinical trials, the sample size is calculated based on the desired effect size and power while controlling the type I error rate. In sequential clinical trials, testing of the primary hypotheses may occur during one or more interim analyses as well as a final analysis. Without proper adjustments, this inflates the trial-wise type I error rate. Appropriate methods are required to maintain its strong control at a pre-specified significance level. Many group sequential methods have been proposed (e.g., Lan and DeMets 1983; O'Brien and Fleming 1979; Pocock 1977, 1997) and are widely used in clinical trials to allow early termination of the trials due to overwhelming efficacy, futility, or undue harm.

As summarized in Table 6.1, several designs and analyses of group sequential clinical trials with multiple endpoints have been proposed.

Asakura et al. (2014a, b) discuss group sequential design in clinical trials with two co-primary endpoints and evaluate how the power and sample sizes behave with varying correlation, information fraction, effect sizes and the type of design (i.e., Pocock, O'Brien-Fleming and their mixed designs). Several authors have discussed procedures with other inferential goals for multiple endpoints in group sequential designs. For the global procedure, Tang et al. (1989) discuss a method based on a generalized

Table 6.1 Summary of designs and analyses of group sequential clinical trials with multiple endpoints

Endpoint scale	Alternative hypothesis	
	Effect on all endpoints	Effect on at least one endpoint
Continuous	Asakura et al. (2014a)	Jennison and Turnbull (1993)
	Jennison and Turnbull (1993)	Kosorok et al. (2004)
		Tamhane et al. (2010, 2012a, b)
		Tang et al. (1989)
		Tang and Geller (1999)
Binary	Asakura et al. (2014b)	
Time-to-event		Kosorok et al. (2004)

least squares procedure by O'Brien (1987). Tang and Geller (1999) discuss a method based on the closed testing procedures, and Tamhane et al. (2010, 2012a, b) consider methods based on the gatekeeping procedures (Dmitrienko and Tamhabe 2007; Demitrienko et al. 2010). Kosorok et al. (2004) discuss group sequential designs with multiple primary endpoints, with use of a global alpha-spending function to control the overall type I error and a multiple decision rule to control error rates for concluding wrong alternative hypotheses. Jennison and Turnbull (1993) describe group sequential tests for a bivariate normal response, where the indifference region approach is adopted.

As an extension of the method discussed in Evans et al. (2007) and Li et al. (2009), by using prediction to convey information regarding potential effect size estimates and associated precision with trial continuation, Evans et al. (2011) discuss "predicted rings" and conditional power contour plots as a flexible and practical strategy for monitoring trials with co-primary (e.g., benefit:risk) endpoints.

Time-to-Event Endpoints

As mentioned in Chap. 1, the ARDENT Study is designed with two co-primary endpoints: time to virologic failure (efficacy endpoint) and time to discontinuation of randomized treatment due to toxicity. For such time-to-events endpoints, Sugimoto et al. (2011, 2012a, 2013) derive a log-rank based method for sample sizing although their research was limited to two time-to-event endpoints and independent censoring. They use typical copula families to model the endpoints, i.e., Clayton copula (Clayton 1978), positive stable copula (Hougaard 1984, 1986) and Frank copula (Frank 1979; Genest 1987). They evaluate how the sample size varies as a function of the correlation between the endpoints, where the study objective is to evaluate the simultaneous effect on both endpoints and for evaluating the effect on at least one endpoint. In addition, Hamasaki et al. (2013) discuss a simpler method for calculating the sample size for two correlated time-to-event endpoints as co-primary when the time-to-event outcomes are exponentially distributed.

Mixed Endpoints

Other trials with co-primary endpoints may have endpoints with mixed scales of measurement. One example of a clinical trial with mixed-scale endpoints as co-primary is the PREMIER study (Breedveld et al. 2006), a trial enrolling participants with early aggressive rheumatoid arthritis. The trial has two co-primary endpoints: (1) ACR50 response (a binary endpoint) and (2) the change from baseline in the modified total Sharp score (mTSS) (a continuous endpoint). Another example is the VALOR trial (Rudnick et al. 2008) which enrolled participants with chronic kidney disease. The trial has two mixed co-primary endpoints: (1) the peak percentage change from baseline serum creatinine over the 72-h period after contrast media administration (a continuous endpoint) and (2) contrast-induced nephropathy defined as an increase of 0.5 mg/dL or more from baseline serum creatinine within 72-h (a binary endpoint). A third example is the ACCENT I trial (Stephen et al. 2002), a trial enrolling participants with active Crohn's disease who receive a single infusion of infliximab to assess the benefit of maintenance infliximab therapy. The trial has two mixed co-primary endpoints: (1) response at week 2 and in remission (Crohn's disease activity index < 150) at week 30 (a binary endpoint), and (2) the time to loss of response up to week 54 in patients who responded.

For mixed continuous and binary co-primary endpoints, the necessary sample size methodology can be developed as an extension of the methods discussed in Chaps. 2 and 3. But there are complexities. One major issue is deciding how to model the relationship between the two endpoints. Several measures or models have been proposed to define the relationship between continuous and binary variables (Dale 1986; Lev 1949; Molenberghs et al. 2001; Pearson 1909; Plackett 1965; Tate 1954). Sozu et al. (2012) discuss sample size methodology assuming that the endpoints are distributed as a multivariate normal distribution, where binary variables are observed in a dichotomized normal distribution with a certain point of dichotomy.

For mixed time-to-event and binary endpoints, Sugimoto et al. (2012b) define the relationship between the endpoints under the limited distributions of copulas. They evaluate how the correlation is restricted depending on the marginal probabilities of binary endpoints, and discuss how the sample size varies as a function of the correlation.

References

Asakura K, Hamasaki , Sugimoto T, Hayashi K, Evans S, Sozu T (2014a) Sample size determination in group-sequential clinical trials with two co-primary endpoints. Stat Med 33:2897–2913

Asakura K, Hamasaki T, Evans SR, Sugimoto T, Sozu T (2014b) Group-sequential designs when considering two binary outcomes as co-primary endpoints. In Chen Z et al (eds) Recent advances in applied statistics. Springer, New York 235–262

Bloch DA, Lai TL, Tubert-Bitter P (2001) One-sided tests in clinical trials with multiple endpoints. Biometrics 57:1039–1047

Breedveld FC, Weisman MH, Kavanaugh AF, Cohen SB, Pavelka K, van Vollenhoven R, Sharp J, Perez JL, Spencer-Green GT (2006) The PREMIER study: a multicenter, randomized, double blind clinical trial of combination therapy with adalimumab plus methotrexate versus methotrexate alone or adalimumab alone in patients with early, aggressive rheumatoid arthritis who had not had previous methotrexate treatment. Arthritis Rheum 51:26–37

Clayton DG (1978) A model for association in bivariate life tables and its application in epidemiological studies of familial tendency in chronic disease. Biometrika 65:141–151

Dale JR (1986) Global cross-ratio models for bivariate, discrete, ordered responses. Biometrics 42:909–917

Dmitrienko A, Tamhane AC, Bretz F (2010) Multiple testing problems in pharmaceutical statistics. Chapman & Hall/CRC, Boca Raton

Dmitrienko A, Tamhabe AC (2007) Gatekeeping procedure with clinical trial applications. J Biopharm Stat 6:171–180

Evans SR, Hamasaki T, Hayashi K (2011) Design and data monitoring of clinical trials with co-primary benefit:risk endpoints using prediction. In: The joint meeting of the (2011) Taipei international statistical symposium and the 7th conference of Asian regional section of the IASC, Taipei, Taiwan, 16–19 Dec

Evans SR, Li L, Wei LJ (2007) Data monitoring in clinical trials using prediction. Drug Inf J 41:733–742

Frank MJ (1979) On the simultaneous associativity of $F(x, y)$ and $x + y - F(x, y)$. Aequationes Math 19:194–226

Genest C (1987) Frank's family of bivariate distribution. Biometrika 74:549–555

Hamasaki T, Sugimoto T, Evans SR, Sozu T (2013) Sample size determination for clinical trials with co-primary outcomes: exponential event-times. Pharm Stat 12:28–34

Hougaard P (1984) Life table methods for heterogeneous populations: distributions describing the heterogeneity. Biometrika 71:75–83

Hougaard P (1986) A class of multivariate failure time distribution. Biometrika 73:671–678

Jennison C, Turnbull BW (1993) Group sequential tests for bivariate response: interim analyses of clinical trials with both efficacy and safety endpoints. Biometrics 49:741–752

Kosorok MR, Shi Y, DeMets DL (2004) Design and analysis of group sequential clinical trials with multiple primary endpoints. Biometrics 60:134–145

Lan KKG, DeMets DL (1983) Discrete sequential boundaries for clinical trials. Biometrika 70:659–663

Lev J (1949) The point biserial coefficient of correlation. Ann Math Stat 20:125–126

Li L, Evans SR, Uno H, Wei LJ (2009) Predicted interval plots (PIPS): a graphical tool for data monitoring of clinical trials. Stat Biopharm Res 1:348–355

Molenberghs G, Geys H, Buyse M (2001) Evaluation of surrogate endpoints in randomized experiments with mixed discrete and continuous outcomes. Stat Med 20:3023–3038

O'Brien PC (1987) Procedure for comparing samples with multiple endpoints. Biometrics 40:1079–1087

O'Brien PC, Fleming TR (1979) A multiple testing procedure for clinical trials. Biometrics 35:549–556

Pearson K (1909) On a new method for determining the correlation between a measured character A, and a character B. Biometrika 7:96–105

Plackett RL (1965) A class of bivariate distributions. J Am Stat Assoc 60:516–522

Pocock SJ (1977) Group sequential methods in the design and analysis of clinical trials. Biometrika 64:191–199

Pocock SJ (1997) Clinical trials with multiple outcomes: a statistical perspective on their design, analysis and interpretation. Control Clin Trials 18:530–545

Röhmel J, Gerlinger C, Benda N, Läuter J (2006) On testing simultaneously non-inferiority in two multiple primary endpoints and superiority in at least one of them. Biometrical J 48:916–933

Rudnick MR, Davidson C, Laskey W, Stafford JL, Sherwin PF (2008) VALOR Trial Investigators. Nephrotoxicity of iodixanol versus ioversol in patients with chronic kidney disease: the Visipaque

Angiography/Interventions with Laboratory Outcomes in Renal Insufficiency (VALOR) Trial. Am Heart J 156:776–782

Sozu T, Sugimoto T, Hamasaki T (2012) Sample size determination in clinical trials with multiple co-primary endpoints including mixed continuous and binary variables. Biometrical J 54:716–729

Stephen B, Hanauer SB, Feagan BG, Lichtenstein GR, Mayer LF, Schreiber S, Colombel JF, Rachmilewitz D, Wolf DC, Olson A, Bao W, Rutgeerts P (2002) The ACCENT I study group. Maintenance infliximab for Crohn's disease: the ACCENT I randomised trial. Lancet 359:1541–1549

Sugimoto T, Hamasaki T, Sozu T (2011) Sample size determination in clinical trials with two correlated co-primary time-to-event endpoints. In: The 7th international conference on multiple comparison procedures, Washington DC, USA, 29 Aug –1 Sept

Sugimoto T, Sozu T, Hamasaki T (2012a) A convenient formula for sample size calculations in clinical trials with multiple co-primary continuous endpoints. Pharm Stat 11:118–128

Sugimoto T, Hamasaki T, Sozu T, Evans SR (2012b) Sample size determination in clinical trials with two correlated time-to-event endpoints as primary contrast. In: The 6th FDA-DIA statistics forum, Washington DC, USA, April 22–25

Sugimoto T, Sozu T, Hamasaki T, Evans SR (2013) A logrank test-based method for sizing clinical trials with two co-primary time-to-events endpoints. Biostatistics 14:409–421

Tamhane AC, Meta CR, Liu L (2010) Testing a primary and a secondary endpoint in a group sequential design. Biometrics 66:1174–1184

Tamhane AC, Wu Y, Mehta CR (2012a) Adaptive extensions of a two-stage group sequential procedure for testing primary and secondary endpoints (I): unknown correlation between the endpoints. Stat Med 31:2027–2040

Tamhane AC, Wu Y, Mehta CR (2012b) Adaptive extensions of a two-stage group sequential procedure for testing primary and secondary endpoints (II): sample size re-estimation. Stat Med 31:2041–2054

Tang DI, Gnecco C, Geller NL (1989) Design of group sequential clinical trials with multiple endpoints. J Am Stat Assoc 84:776–779

Tang DI, Geller NL (1999) Closed testing procedures for group sequential clinical trials with multiple endpoints. Biometrics 55:1188–1192

Tate RF (1954) Correlation between a discrete and a continuous variable. Point-biserial correlation. Ann Math Stat 25:603–607

Appendix A
Sample Size Calculation Using Other
Contrasts for Binary Endpoints

Chapter 3 provided methods for power and sample size determination when the alternative hypothesis is joint differences in proportions for all binary endpoints. The two other measures for binary endpoints, the risk ratio $\psi_k = \pi_{Tk}/\pi_{Ck}$ and the odds ratio $\varphi_k = (\pi_{Tk}\theta_{Ck})/(\theta_{Tk}\pi_{Ck})$, are also used in clinical trials, where $\theta_{Tk} = 1 - \pi_{Tk}$ and $\theta_{Ck} = 1 - \pi_{Ck}$. In this appendix, we outline the sample size methodology for clinical trials with multiple risk ratios and odds ratios as primary contrasts.

A.1 Risk Ratio

Consider a randomized clinical trial comparing two interventions with K binary endpoints. By analogy to the sample size method for a single endpoint (e.g., Wood 1992; Sahai and Khurshid 1996) to evaluate simultaneous reduction effects on the occurrence of events, one straightforward approach is to test the null hypothesis $H_0 : \pi_{Tk} - \pi_{Ck} \geq 0$ for at least one k versus the alternative hypothesis $H_1 : \pi_{Tk}/\pi_{Ck} < 1$ for all k, at significance level of α. The well-known test statistics for this situation are the test statistics in (3.1) in Chap. 3. The same sample size methodology can be used for the multiple risk ratios.

An alternative method is based on the asymptotic distribution of the log-transformed risk ratios. As a consequence of the delta method, for large sample size, it is well known that the natural logarithm of an observed proportion, $\log p_{Tk}$ and $\log p_{Ck}$ are approximately normally distributed as

$$N\left(\log \pi_{Tk}, \theta_{Tk}/(n_T \pi_{Tk})\right) \quad \text{and} \quad N\left(\log \pi_{Ck}, \theta_{Ck}/(n_C \pi_{Ck})\right)$$

respectively (e.g., Lachin 2011). Therefore, to detect the superiority for ALL K log-transformed risk ratios, we test the null hypothesis $H_0 : \log \psi_k \geq 0$ for at least one k versus the alternative hypothesis $H_0 : \log \psi_k < 0$ for all K at a significance level of α.

© The Author(s) 2015
T. Sozu et al., *Sample Size Determination in Clinical Trials with Multiple Endpoints*,
SpringerBriefs in Statistics, DOI 10.1007/978-3-319-22005-5

We have the K log-transformed (observed) risk ratios $\log R_k = \log(p_{Tk}/p_{Ck})$ $(k = 1, \ldots, K)$. For large sample size, the distribution of the vector of $(\log R_1, \ldots, \log R_K)^{\mathrm{T}}$ is approximately K-variate normal with mean vector $\boldsymbol{\mu} = (\log \psi_1, \ldots, \log \psi_K)^{\mathrm{T}}$ and covariance matrix $\boldsymbol{\Sigma}$ determined by

$$
\begin{cases}
\sigma_k^2 = \dfrac{1}{n}\left(\dfrac{\theta_{Tk}}{\pi_{Tk}} + \dfrac{\theta_{Ck}}{\pi_{Ck}}\left(\dfrac{1-\kappa}{\kappa}\right)\right) & k = k' \\[2ex]
\sigma_{kk'} = \dfrac{1}{n}\left(\tau_T^{kk'}\dfrac{\sqrt{\theta_{Tk}\theta_{Tk'}}}{\sqrt{\pi_{Tk}\pi_{Tk'}}} + \tau_C^{kk'}\dfrac{\sqrt{\theta_{Ck}\theta_{Ck'}}}{\sqrt{\pi_{Ck}\pi_{Ck'}}}\left(\dfrac{1-\kappa}{\kappa}\right)\right) & k \neq k'.
\end{cases}
$$

Therefore, the correlation between the risk ratios, $\rho_R^{kk'} = \mathrm{corr}[\log R_k, \log R_{k'}]$ is approximately given by

$$
\rho_R^{kk'} = \frac{\kappa\tau_T^{kk'}\sqrt{\theta_{Tk}\theta_{Tk'}\pi_{Ck}\pi_{Ck'}} + (1-\kappa)\tau_C^{kk'}\sqrt{\pi_{Tk}\pi_{Tk'}\theta_{Ck}\theta_{Ck'}}}{\sqrt{(\kappa\theta_{Tk}\pi_{Ck} + (1-\kappa)\pi_{Tk}\theta_{Ck})(\kappa\theta_{Tk'}\pi_{Ck'} + (1-\kappa)\pi_{Tk'}\theta_{Ck'})}}.
$$

If the correlation between endpoints is assumed to be common between the two groups, i.e., $\tau_T^{kk'} = \tau_C^{kk'} = \tau^{kk'}$, then we have

$$
\rho_R^{kk'} = \frac{\tau^{kk'} A}{\sqrt{A^2 + \kappa(1-\kappa)B^2}},
$$

where

$$
A = \kappa\sqrt{\theta_{Tk}\theta_{Tk'}\pi_{Ck}\pi_{Ck'}} + (1-\kappa)\sqrt{\pi_{Tk}\pi_{Tk'}\theta_{Ck}\theta_{Ck'}}
$$

and

$$
B = \sqrt{\theta_{Tk}\pi_{Tk'}\pi_{Ck}\theta_{Ck'}} - \sqrt{\pi_{Tk}\theta_{Tk'}\theta_{Ck}\pi_{Ck'}}.
$$

Clearly $|\rho_R^{kk'}| \leq \tau^{kk'}$ and $\rho_R^{kk'} = \tau^{kk'}$ when $\tau^{kk'} = 0$, or $\pi_{Tk}/\theta_{Tk} = \pi_{Tk'}/\theta_{Tk'}$. Hereafter, we simply assume a common correlation between the two groups.

Let Z_k be the test statistics for the log-transformed risk ratio $\log \psi_k$ given by

$$
Z_k = \log R_k \bigg/ \sqrt{\frac{\bar{q}_k}{\kappa n \bar{p}_k}}
$$

where $\bar{p}_k = (1-\kappa)p_{Tk} + \kappa p_{Ck}$ and $\bar{q}_k = 1 - \bar{p}_k$. When H_1 is joint effects on ALL risk ratios, the hypotheses for testing $H_0 : \log \psi \geq 0$ for at least one k versus $H_1 : \log \psi < 0$ for all k are tested using the test statistics $(Z_1, \ldots, Z_K)$. The rejection region of H_0 is $[\{Z_1 < -z_\alpha\} \cap \cdots \cap \{Z_K < -z_\alpha\}]$. Therefore, for the risk ratios

ψ_k, for large sample size, straightforward algebra and substitution of population parameters for estimates provides the approximate overall power of

$$1 - \beta = \Pr\left[\bigcap_{k=1}^{K} \{Z_k < -z_\alpha\} \,\bigg|\, H_1\right] \simeq \Pr\left[\bigcap_{k=1}^{K} \{Z_k^* < c_k^*\} \,\bigg|\, H_1\right], \qquad (A.1)$$

where

$$Z_k^* = (\log R_k - \log \psi_k)\bigg/ \sqrt{\frac{1}{n}\left(\frac{\theta_{Tk}}{\pi_{Tk}} + \frac{\theta_{Ck}}{\pi_{Ck}}\left(\frac{1-\kappa}{\kappa}\right)\right)},$$

$$c_k^* = -\left(z_\alpha\sqrt{\frac{\bar{\theta}_k}{\kappa n \bar{\pi}_k}} + \log \psi_k\right)\bigg/ \sqrt{\frac{1}{n}\left(\frac{\theta_{Tk}}{\pi_{Tk}} + \frac{\theta_{Ck}}{\pi_{Ck}}\left(\frac{1-\kappa}{\kappa}\right)\right)},$$

$\bar{\pi}_k = (1-\kappa)\pi_{Tk} + \kappa\pi_{Ck}$ and $\bar{\theta}_k = 1 - \bar{\pi}_k$. The overall power (1.1) is calculated by using $\Phi_K(-c_1^*, \ldots, -c_K^*)$, where Φ_K is the cumulative distribution function of $N_K(\mathbf{0}, \rho_Z)$; the off-diagonal element of the correlation matrix ρ_Z is given by $\rho_{Z*}^{kk'} = \rho_R^{kk'}$.

The sample size required to detect the superiority for all of the risk ratios with the overall power $1 - \beta$ at a significance level of α is the smallest integer not less than n satisfying $1 - \beta \leq \Phi_K(-c_1^*, \ldots, -c_K^*)$. The required sample size can be simplified to improve the approximation to normality as it is known that

$$\frac{q_{Tk}}{p_{Tk}} + \frac{q_{Ck}}{p_{Ck}}\left(\frac{1-\kappa}{\kappa}\right) \geq \frac{\bar{q}_k}{\kappa \bar{p}_k}.$$

If we assume a un-pooled variance under the alternative hypothesis, we have

$$\dot{c}_k^* = -z_\alpha - \log \psi_k \bigg/ \sqrt{\frac{1}{n}\left(\frac{\theta_{Tk}}{\pi_{Tk}} + \frac{\theta_{Ck}}{\pi_{Ck}}\left(\frac{1-\kappa}{\kappa}\right)\right)}.$$

So that the sample size required to achieve the desired power $1 - \beta$ is the smallest integer not less than n satisfying $1 - \beta \leq \Phi_K(-\dot{c}_1^*, \ldots, -\dot{c}_K^*)$. This sample size will be relatively larger than the sample size satisfying $1 - \beta \leq \Phi_K(-c_1^*, \ldots, -c_K^*)$, but this may lead to the improvement of the approximation, by analogy with sample size determination for a single risk ratio.

In our experience (Hamasaki et al. 2011, 2012), the asymptotic normal approximation method may work well in most situations, except for a situation where $\psi_k \geq 0.5$ and π_{Ck} is so close to zero (or one). In this situation, use of the method assuming a un-pooled variance under the alternative hypothesis is recommended.

A.2 Odds Ratio

We outline a method for the calculation of the sample size to detect the superiority for ALL K odds ratios. We now have K log-transformed (observed) odds ratios $\log O_k$ where $O_k = (p_{Tk}q_{Ck})/(q_{Tk}p_{Ck})$. For large sample size, as a conquence of delta method, the distribution of the vector of $(\log O_1, \ldots, \log O_K)^{\mathrm{T}}$ is approximately K-variate normal with mean vector $\mu = (\log \varphi_1, \ldots, \log \varphi_K)^{\mathrm{T}}$ and covariance matrix Σ determined by

$$
\begin{cases}
\sigma_k^2 = \dfrac{1}{n}\left(\dfrac{1}{\pi_{Tk}\theta_{Tk}} + \dfrac{1}{\pi_{Ck}\theta_{Ck}}\left(\dfrac{1-\kappa}{\kappa}\right)\right) & k = k' \\[3mm]
\sigma_{kk'} = \dfrac{1}{n}\left(\dfrac{\tau_T^{kk'}}{\sqrt{\pi_{Tk}\theta_{Tk}\pi_{Tk'}\theta_{Tk'}}} + \dfrac{\tau_C^{kk'}}{\sqrt{\pi_{Ck}\theta_{Ck}\pi_{Ck'}\theta_{Ck'}}}\left(\dfrac{1-\kappa}{\kappa}\right)\right) & k \neq k'.
\end{cases}
$$

where $\varphi_k = (\pi_{Tk}\theta_{Ck})/(\theta_{Tk}\pi_{Ck})$. Therefore, the correlation between the log-transformed odds ratios, $\rho_O^{kk'} = \mathrm{corr}[\log O_k, \log O_{k'}]$ is given by

$$
\rho_O^{kk'} = \frac{\kappa\tau_T^{kk'}\sqrt{\pi_{Ck}\theta_{Ck}\pi_{Ck'}\theta_{Ck'}} + (1-\kappa)\tau_C^{kk'}\sqrt{\pi_{Tk}\theta_{Tk}\pi_{Tk'}\theta_{Tk'}}}{\sqrt{(\kappa\pi_{Ck}\theta_{Ck} + (1-\kappa)\pi_{Tk}\theta_{Tk})(\kappa\pi_{Ck'}\theta_{Ck'} + (1-\kappa)\pi_{Tk'}\theta_{Tk'})}}.
$$

Let Z_k be the test statistics for the log-transformed odds ratios $\log \varphi_k$, given by

$$
Z_k = \log O_k \Big/ \sqrt{\frac{1}{\kappa n \bar{\pi}_k \bar{\theta}_k}} \quad (k = 1, \ldots, K).
$$

When evaluating joint effects on all of the correlated odds ratios, the hypotheses for testing $H_0 : \log \varphi_k \geq 0$ for at least one k versus $H_1 : \log \varphi_k < 0$ for all k, are tested by the above test statistics $(Z_1, \ldots, Z_K)$. The rejection region of H_0 is $[\{Z_1 < -z_\alpha\} \cap \cdots \cap \{Z_K < -z_\alpha\}]$. Therefore, for the odds ratios φ_k, the overall power is given by

$$
1 - \beta = \Pr\left[\bigcap_{k=1}^{K}\{Z_k < -z_\alpha\} \,\Big|\, H_1\right]
$$

$$
\simeq \Pr\left[\bigcap_{k=1}^{K}\left\{\frac{\log O_k - \log \varphi_k}{\dfrac{1}{n}\left(\dfrac{1}{\pi_{Tk}\theta_{Tk}} + \dfrac{1}{\pi_{Ck}\theta_{Ck}}\left(\dfrac{1-\kappa}{\kappa}\right)\right)} < c_k\right\} \,\Big|\, H_1\right], \quad (A.2)
$$

where

$$
c_k = -\left(z_\alpha\sqrt{\frac{1}{\kappa n \bar{\pi}_k \bar{\theta}_k}} + \log \varphi_k\right)\Big/ \sqrt{\frac{1}{n}\left(\frac{1}{\pi_{Tk}\theta_{Tk}} + \frac{1}{\pi_{Ck}\theta_{Ck}}\left(\frac{1-\kappa}{\kappa}\right)\right)}.
$$

The overall power is calculated by using $\Phi_K(-c_1^*, \ldots, -c_K^*)$.

The sample size required to detect the superiority for all of the odds ratios with the overall power $1 - \beta$ at a significance level of α is the smallest integer not less than n satisfying $1 - \beta \leq \Phi_K(-c_1^*, \ldots, -c_K^*)$. Similarly, if we assume a un-pooled variance under the alternative hypothesis, we have a simplified

$$c_k' = -z_\alpha - \log \varphi_k \bigg/ \sqrt{\frac{1}{n}\left(\frac{1}{\pi_{Tk}\theta_{Tk}} + \frac{1}{\pi_{Ck}\theta_{Ck}}\left(\frac{1-\kappa}{\kappa}\right)\right)}.$$

The sample size required to achieve the desired power $1 - \beta$ is given by the smallest integer not less than n satisfying $1 - \beta \leq \Phi(-c_1', \ldots, -c_K')$.

References

Hamasaki T, Evans SR, Sugimoto T, Sozu T (2011) Power and sample size determination for clinical trials with two correlated binary relative risks. In: The 2011 international conference on applied statistics, 26–27 May 2011, Taipei, Taiwan

Hamasaki T, Evans SR, Sugimoto T, Sozu T (2012) Power and sample size determination for clinical trials with two correlated binary relative risks. In: ENAR Spring Meeting 2012, 1–4 April 2012, Washington DC, USA

Lachin JM (2011) Biostatistical methods: the asssessment of relative risks, 2nd edn. Wiley, New York

Sahai H, Khurshid A (1996) Formulae and tables for the determination of sample sizes and power in clinical trials for testing differences in proportions for the two-sample design: a review. Stat. Med. 15:1–21

Wood M (1992) Formulae for sample size, power and minimum detecable relative risk in medical studies. Statistician 41:185–196

Appendix B
Empirical Power for Sample Size Calculation for Binary Co-primary Endpoints

As mentioned in Sect. 3.2.2, there are more direct approaches for sample size calculation without using an asymptotic normal approximation, however, such methods are computationally difficult and often impractical, particularly for the large sample sizes. On the other hand, the methodology using the asymptotic normal approximation discussed in Sect. 3.2.1 may not work well when events are rare or when sample sizes are small. We performed a Monte-Carlo simulation study and computed the empirical powers for the corresponding test and the Fisher's exact test in order to evaluate the utility of the continuity correction and/or the arcsine root transformation for the test statistics. By using the method described in Emrich and Piedmonte (1991), we generated random numbers Y_{Tjk} and Y_{Cjk}, which are independently multivariate Bernoulli distributed with probabilities of π_{Tk} and π_{Ck}, but the observations within pairs for the two interventions are correlated with a common correlation, i.e., $\rho^{kk'} = \mathrm{corr}[Y_{Tjk}, Y_{Tjk'}] = \mathrm{corr}[Y_{Cjk}, Y_{Cjk'}]$. We conducted 100,000 replications to compute the empirical power for the corresponding test and Fisher's exact test under the sample size calculated by each method with the equal correlation of the multivariate Bernoulli distribution between the endpoints, i.e., $\tau = \tau^{12} = \cdots = \tau^{K-1,K}$ from 0.0 to 0.95 by 0.05 and 0.99. In addition, equal sample sizes per group $n = n_T = n_C$ (i.e., $r = 1.0$) were calculated to detect the joint differences in the proportions between the two interventions with the overall power of $1 - \beta = 0.80$ at the significance level of $\alpha = 0.025$. Figures B.1, B.2, B.3 and B.4 illustrate the behavior of the empirical power for $\tau = 0.0$ and 0.8 as a function of the standardized effect size in the cases of $K = 2$ and 3, where $\pi_{Ck} + 0.05 \leq \pi_{Tk} < 0.95$ by 0.05 with $\pi_{T1} = \cdots = \pi_{TK} = \pi_T$ and $\pi_{C1} = \cdots = \pi_{CK} = \pi_C = 0.5, 0.6, 0.7$ and 0.8.

The chi-square method (without CC) attains the targeted power of 0.8 when the standardized effect size is small. The empirical power is larger than 0.8 as the standardized effect size increases and π_C goes from 0.5 to 0.8, i.e. the required sample size is smaller. The empirical power for the Fisher's exact test is always smaller than 0.8, and it decreases as the standardized effect size increases.

A similar behavior of the empirical power was observed in the chi-square method with CC. When the standardized effect size is small, the chi-square method with CC attains the targeted power of 0.8. The empirical power is larger than 0.8 as the

© The Author(s) 2015
T. Sozu et al., *Sample Size Determination in Clinical Trials with Multiple Endpoints*,
SpringerBriefs in Statistics, DOI 10.1007/978-3-319-22005-5

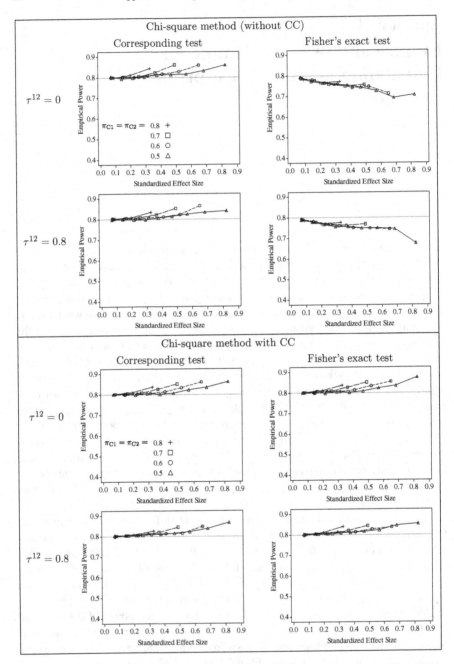

Fig. B.1 Empirical power for the chi-square methods with and without CC for two co-primary binary endpoints ($K = 2$) with the desired overall power of $1 - \beta = 0.80$

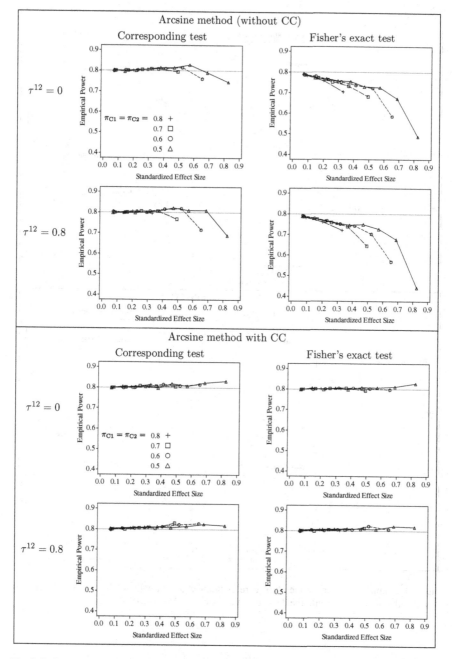

Fig. B.2 Empirical power for the arcsine methods with and without CC for two co-primary binary endpoints ($K = 2$) with the desired overall power of $1 - \beta = 0.80$

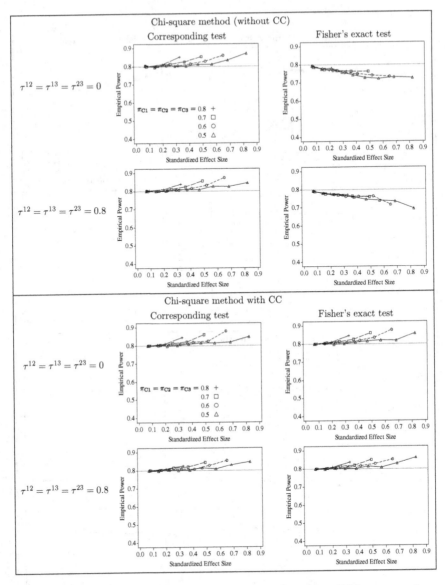

Fig. B.3 Empirical power for the chi-square methods with and without CC for two co-primary binary endpoints ($K = 2$) with the desired overall power of $1 - \beta = 0.80$

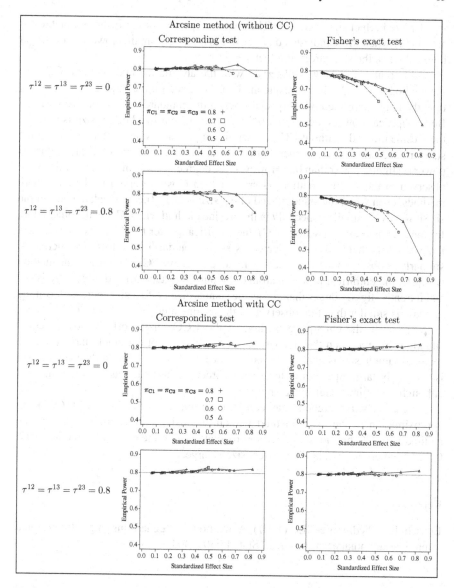

Fig. B.4 Empirical power for the arcsine methods with and without CC for two co-primary binary endpoints ($K = 2$) with the desired overall power of $1 - \beta = 0.80$

standardized effect size increases. The empirical power for the Fisher's exact test is around 0.8 when the standardized effect size is relatively small. However, it is larger than 0.8 when the standardized effect size is larger.

A different behavior was observed with the arcsine method (without CC) and the method with CC. These arcsine methods better attain the targeted power of 0.8 than the chi-square methods, especially when the standardized effect size is small. Both empirical powers are around 0.8 until the standardized effect size is 0.5. For the arcsine method (without CC), the empirical power is smaller than 0.8 when the standardized effect size is larger, but for the arcsine method with CC the empirical power is slightly larger than 0.8. However, the degree of such an increase or decrease observed in the arcsine methods is smaller than those observed in the chi-square methods, even when the standardized effect size is large (i.e., the calculated sample size is relatively small), especially in the arcsine method with CC. On the other hand, for the arcsine method (without CC), the empirical power for the Fisher's exact test is always less than 0.8 and it decreases as the standardized effect size increases, similarly as observed in the chi-square method (without CC). For the arcsine method with CC, the empirical power is around 0.8 until the standardized effect size is 0.5 and it trends slightly larger than 0.8 as the standardized effect size increases. But the increase is smaller than that observed in the arcsine method (without CC).

As a result, the chi-square method (without CC) may work in most practical situations except when the standardized effect size is not extremely large (i.e., the required sample size is relatively small). However, when the standardized effect size is extremely large, it is better to use any direct method such as the exact method although it requires extensive computations.

Alternatively, researchers may consider the use of the methods with CC as an approximation to the exact method without extensive computations. The arcsine method with CC provides a better approximation than the chi-square method with CC even when the standardized effect size is large.

Reference

Emrich LJ, Piedmonte MR (1991) A method for generating high-dimensional multivariate binary variates. Am. Stat. 45:302–304

Appendix C
Numerical Tables for C_k in the Convenient Sample Size Formula for the Three Co-primary Continuous Endpoints

See Tables C.1, C.2.

© The Author(s) 2015
T. Sozu et al., *Sample Size Determination in Clinical Trials with Multiple Endpoints*,
SpringerBriefs in Statistics, DOI 10.1007/978-3-319-22005-5

Table C.1 $C_K(\beta, \rho, \gamma, \alpha)$ when $1-\beta = 0.8$, $\alpha = 0.025$ and $K = 3$, where $\gamma = (\gamma_1, \gamma_2) = (\delta_1/\delta_3, \delta_2/\delta_3)$, H = 0.8, M = 0.5, and L = 0.3

$\rho = \begin{pmatrix} 1 & & \\ M & 1 & \\ M & M & 1 \end{pmatrix}$ $\begin{pmatrix} 1 & & \\ H & 1 & \\ H & H & 1 \end{pmatrix}$

γ_2 \ γ_1	1.0	1.1	1.2	1.3	1.4	1.5	2.0	
1.0	1.182	1.109	1.079	1.069	1.067	1.066	1.066	1.0
2.0	0.842	1.016	0.973	0.956	0.951	0.950	0.950	1.1
1.5	0.855	0.866	0.920	0.898	0.890	0.888	0.887	1.2
1.4	0.871	0.881	0.895	0.871	0.862	0.859	0.858	1.3
1.3	0.902	0.910	0.922	0.946	0.851	0.848	0.847	1.4
1.2	0.955	0.961	0.970	0.990	1.029	0.844	0.843	1.5
1.1	1.040	1.043	1.050	1.065	1.096	1.155	0.842	2.0
1.0	1.168	1.170	1.174	1.184	1.207	1.254	1.339	γ_2
	2.0	1.5	1.4	1.3	1.2	1.1	1.0	γ_1

$\begin{pmatrix} 1 & & \\ 0 & 1 & \\ 0 & 0 & 1 \end{pmatrix}$ $\begin{pmatrix} 1 & & \\ L & 1 & \\ L & L & 1 \end{pmatrix}$

γ_2 \ γ_1	1.0	1.1	1.2	1.3	1.4	1.5	2.0	
1.0	1.402	1.314	1.261	1.233	1.219	1.213	1.210	1.0
2.0	0.842	1.212	1.149	1.112	1.093	1.083	1.077	1.1
1.5	0.874	0.900	1.077	1.033	1.008	0.995	0.986	1.2
1.4	0.903	0.926	0.948	0.983	0.954	0.938	0.925	1.3
1.3	0.948	0.967	0.987	1.021	0.921	0.903	0.886	1.4
1.2	1.016	1.030	1.046	1.076	1.124	0.882	0.864	1.5
1.1	1.114	1.123	1.135	1.159	1.200	1.268	0.842	2.0
1.0	1.250	1.256	1.264	1.281	1.314	1.371	1.463	γ_2
	2.0	1.5	1.4	1.3	1.2	1.1	1.0	γ_1

$\begin{pmatrix} 1 & & \\ M & 1 & \\ H & H & 1 \end{pmatrix}$ $\begin{pmatrix} 1 & & \\ H & 1 & \\ H & M & 1 \end{pmatrix}$

γ_2 \ γ_1	1.0	1.1	1.2	1.3	1.4	1.5	2.0	
1.0	1.230	1.183	1.171	1.169	1.168	1.168	1.168	1.0
2.0	0.842	1.069	1.046	1.041	1.040	1.040	1.040	1.1
1.5	0.843	0.844	0.968	0.957	0.955	0.955	0.955	1.2
1.4	0.847	0.848	0.851	0.907	0.903	0.902	0.902	1.3
1.3	0.858	0.859	0.863	0.873	0.873	0.871	0.871	1.4
1.2	0.887	0.888	0.891	0.901	0.927	0.855	0.855	1.5
1.1	0.950	0.951	0.953	0.962	0.985	1.037	0.842	2.0
1.0	1.066	1.067	1.068	1.075	1.093	1.139	1.230	γ_2
	2.0	1.5	1.4	1.3	1.2	1.1	1.0	γ_1

$\begin{pmatrix} 1 & & \\ L & 1 & \\ H & H & 1 \end{pmatrix}$ $\begin{pmatrix} 1 & & \\ H & 1 & \\ H & L & 1 \end{pmatrix}$

γ_2 \ γ_1	1.0	1.1	1.2	1.3	1.4	1.5	2.0	
1.0	1.240	1.211	1.210	1.210	1.210	1.210	1.210	1.0
2.0	0.842	1.085	1.077	1.077	1.077	1.077	1.077	1.1
1.5	0.843	0.844	0.987	0.986	0.986	0.986	0.986	1.2
1.4	0.847	0.848	0.851	0.925	0.925	0.925	0.925	1.3
1.3	0.858	0.859	0.863	0.873	0.886	0.886	0.886	1.4
1.2	0.887	0.888	0.891	0.901	0.928	0.864	0.864	1.5
1.1	0.950	0.951	0.953	0.962	0.985	1.039	0.842	2.0
1.0	1.066	1.067	1.068	1.075	1.095	1.143	1.240	γ_2
	2.0	1.5	1.4	1.3	1.2	1.1	1.0	γ_1

$\begin{pmatrix} 1 & & \\ H & 1 & \\ M & M & 1 \end{pmatrix}$ $\begin{pmatrix} 1 & & \\ M & 1 & \\ M & H & 1 \end{pmatrix}$

γ_2 \ γ_1	1.0	1.1	1.2	1.3	1.4	1.5	2.0	
1.0	1.285	1.185	1.125	1.093	1.077	1.070	1.066	1.0
2.0	0.842	1.101	1.030	0.989	0.967	0.957	0.950	1.1
1.5	0.855	0.863	0.984	0.937	0.910	0.897	0.887	1.2
1.4	0.871	0.877	0.889	0.914	0.885	0.870	0.858	1.3
1.3	0.902	0.906	0.914	0.934	0.875	0.859	0.847	1.4
1.2	0.955	0.957	0.962	0.975	1.007	0.856	0.843	1.5
1.1	1.040	1.040	1.042	1.050	1.071	1.120	0.842	2.0
1.0	1.168	1.169	1.169	1.172	1.183	1.214	1.285	γ_2
	2.0	1.5	1.4	1.3	1.2	1.1	1.0	γ_1

(continued)

Table C.1 (continued)

$\rho = \begin{pmatrix} 1 & & \\ L & 1 & \\ M & M & 1 \end{pmatrix}$
$\begin{pmatrix} 1 & & \\ M & 1 & \\ M & L & 1 \end{pmatrix}$

γ_1	1.0	1.1	1.2	1.3	1.4	1.5	2.0	
γ_2	1.359	1.282	1.241	1.222	1.214	1.211	1.210	1.0
2.0	0.842	1.176	1.124	1.097	1.084	1.079	1.077	1.1
1.5	0.855	0.867	1.049	1.014	0.997	0.990	0.986	1.2
1.4	0.871	0.882	0.896	0.963	0.941	0.931	0.925	1.3
1.3	0.902	0.911	0.924	0.949	0.907	0.895	0.886	1.4
1.2	0.955	0.962	0.973	0.995	1.036	0.874	0.864	1.5
1.1	1.040	1.045	1.053	1.070	1.105	1.167	0.842	2.0
1.0	1.168	1.171	1.177	1.190	1.217	1.269	1.359	γ_2
	2.0	1.5	1.4	1.3	1.2	1.1	1.0	γ_1

$\begin{pmatrix} 1 & & \\ H & 1 & \\ L & L & 1 \end{pmatrix}$
$\begin{pmatrix} 1 & & \\ L & 1 & \\ L & H & 1 \end{pmatrix}$

γ_1	1.0	1.1	1.2	1.3	1.4	1.5	2.0	
γ_2	1.326	1.218	1.149	1.108	1.085	1.074	1.066	1.0
2.0	0.842	1.137	1.058	1.008	0.979	0.963	0.950	1.1
1.5	0.864	0.877	1.013	0.958	0.924	0.905	0.888	1.2
1.4	0.886	0.895	0.909	0.936	0.899	0.878	0.858	1.3
1.3	0.925	0.929	0.939	0.963	0.890	0.868	0.847	1.4
1.2	0.986	0.988	0.993	1.009	1.043	0.865	0.843	1.5
1.1	1.077	1.078	1.080	1.088	1.110	1.160	0.842	2.0
1.0	1.210	1.210	1.211	1.214	1.225	1.256	1.326	γ_2
	2.0	1.5	1.4	1.3	1.2	1.1	1.0	γ_1

$\begin{pmatrix} 1 & & \\ M & 1 & \\ L & L & 1 \end{pmatrix}$
$\begin{pmatrix} 1 & & \\ L & 1 & \\ L & M & 1 \end{pmatrix}$

γ_1	1.0	1.1	1.2	1.3	1.4	1.5	2.0	
γ_2	1.381	1.286	1.229	1.197	1.180	1.173	1.168	1.0
2.0	0.842	1.190	1.122	1.081	1.059	1.048	1.040	1.1
1.5	0.864	0.881	1.057	1.009	0.982	0.967	0.955	1.2
1.4	0.886	0.901	0.918	0.967	0.935	0.917	0.902	1.3
1.3	0.925	0.936	0.950	0.978	0.909	0.889	0.871	1.4
1.2	0.986	0.993	1.004	1.027	1.068	0.875	0.855	1.5
1.1	1.077	1.081	1.089	1.105	1.138	1.198	0.842	2.0
1.0	1.210	1.212	1.216	1.227	1.250	1.297	1.381	γ_2
	2.0	1.5	1.4	1.3	1.2	1.1	1.0	γ_1

$\begin{pmatrix} 1 & & \\ 0 & 1 & \\ M & M & 1 \end{pmatrix}$
$\begin{pmatrix} 1 & & \\ M & 1 & \\ M & 0 & 1 \end{pmatrix}$

γ_1	1.0	1.1	1.2	1.3	1.4	1.5	2.0	
γ_2	1.377	1.307	1.273	1.258	1.253	1.251	1.250	1.0
2.0	0.842	1.196	1.150	1.128	1.119	1.115	1.114	1.1
1.5	0.855	0.867	1.068	1.038	1.025	1.019	1.016	1.2
1.4	0.871	0.882	0.897	0.979	0.961	0.953	0.948	1.3
1.3	0.902	0.912	0.925	0.951	0.919	0.909	0.902	1.4
1.2	0.955	0.963	0.974	0.998	1.041	0.882	0.874	1.5
1.1	1.040	1.045	1.054	1.074	1.111	1.176	0.842	2.0
1.0	1.168	1.172	1.178	1.193	1.225	1.282	1.377	γ_2
	2.0	1.5	1.4	1.3	1.2	1.1	1.0	γ_1

$\begin{pmatrix} 1 & & \\ 0 & 1 & \\ L & L & 1 \end{pmatrix}$
$\begin{pmatrix} 1 & & \\ L & 1 & \\ L & 0 & 1 \end{pmatrix}$

γ_1	1.0	1.1	1.2	1.3	1.4	1.5	2.0	
γ_2	1.422	1.340	1.293	1.269	1.258	1.253	1.250	1.0
2.0	0.842	1.233	1.175	1.143	1.126	1.119	1.114	1.1
1.5	0.864	0.883	1.097	1.057	1.035	1.024	1.016	1.2
1.4	0.886	0.903	0.922	1.000	0.973	0.959	0.948	1.3
1.3	0.925	0.939	0.956	0.987	0.934	0.917	0.903	1.4
1.2	0.986	0.997	1.011	1.038	1.084	0.891	0.874	1.5
1.1	1.077	1.085	1.096	1.118	1.158	1.224	0.842	2.0
1.0	1.210	1.214	1.222	1.239	1.271	1.329	1.422	γ_2
	2.0	1.5	1.4	1.3	1.2	1.1	1.0	γ_1

Table C.2 $C_K(\beta, \rho, \gamma, \alpha)$ when $1 - \beta = 0.9$, $\alpha = 0.025$ and $K = 3$, where $\gamma = (\gamma_1, \gamma_2) = (\delta_1/\delta_3, \delta_2/\delta_3)$, $H = 0.8$, $M = 0.5$, and $L = 0.3$

$\rho =$ $\begin{pmatrix} 1 & & \\ M & 1 & \\ M & M & 1 \end{pmatrix}$

γ_1	1.0	1.1	1.2	1.3	1.4	1.5	2.0	
γ_2	1.603	1.526	1.500	1.494	1.493	1.493	1.493	1.0
2.0	1.282	1.422	1.382	1.370	1.368	1.367	1.367	1.1
1.5	1.285	1.289	1.331	1.315	1.311	1.310	1.310	1.2
1.4	1.293	1.296	1.304	1.295	1.290	1.289	1.289	1.3
1.3	1.313	1.316	1.322	1.339	1.284	1.283	1.283	1.4
1.2	1.356	1.358	1.363	1.377	1.409	1.282	1.282	1.5
1.1	1.437	1.439	1.442	1.452	1.477	1.534	1.282	2.0
1.0	1.577	1.577	1.579	1.585	1.602	1.644	1.734	γ_2
	2.0	1.5	1.4	1.3	1.2	1.1	1.0	γ_1

$\begin{pmatrix} 1 & & \\ H & 1 & \\ H & H & 1 \end{pmatrix}$

$\begin{pmatrix} 1 & & \\ 0 & 1 & \\ 0 & 0 & 1 \end{pmatrix}$

γ_1	1.0	1.1	1.2	1.3	1.4	1.5	2.0	
γ_2	1.780	1.687	1.639	1.618	1.610	1.608	1.607	1.0
2.0	1.282	1.575	1.513	1.483	1.470	1.466	1.463	1.1
1.5	1.291	1.299	1.441	1.403	1.386	1.379	1.375	1.2
1.4	1.305	1.313	1.326	1.360	1.339	1.330	1.325	1.3
1.3	1.336	1.342	1.353	1.378	1.315	1.305	1.299	1.4
1.2	1.392	1.396	1.405	1.426	1.467	1.294	1.288	1.5
1.1	1.486	1.488	1.495	1.510	1.543	1.609	1.282	2.0
1.0	1.632	1.634	1.637	1.647	1.671	1.722	1.818	γ_2
	2.0	1.5	1.4	1.3	1.2	1.1	1.0	γ_1

$\begin{pmatrix} 1 & & \\ L & 1 & \\ L & L & 1 \end{pmatrix}$

$\begin{pmatrix} 1 & & \\ M & 1 & \\ H & H & 1 \end{pmatrix}$

γ_1	1.0	1.1	1.2	1.3	1.4	1.5	2.0	
γ_2	1.642	1.589	1.578	1.577	1.577	1.577	1.577	1.0
2.0	1.282	1.465	1.442	1.438	1.437	1.437	1.437	1.1
1.5	1.282	1.282	1.366	1.357	1.356	1.356	1.356	1.2
1.4	1.283	1.283	1.284	1.316	1.313	1.313	1.313	1.3
1.3	1.289	1.289	1.290	1.296	1.294	1.293	1.293	1.4
1.2	1.310	1.310	1.311	1.316	1.335	1.285	1.285	1.5
1.1	1.367	1.367	1.368	1.372	1.388	1.437	1.282	2.0
1.0	1.493	1.493	1.494	1.496	1.509	1.547	1.642	γ_2
	2.0	1.5	1.4	1.3	1.2	1.1	1.0	γ_1

$\begin{pmatrix} 1 & & \\ H & 1 & \\ H & M & 1 \end{pmatrix}$

$\begin{pmatrix} 1 & & \\ L & 1 & \\ H & H & 1 \end{pmatrix}$

γ_1	1.0	1.1	1.2	1.3	1.4	1.5	2.0	
γ_2	1.647	1.609	1.607	1.607	1.607	1.607	1.607	1.0
2.0	1.282	1.475	1.464	1.463	1.463	1.463	1.463	1.1
1.5	1.282	1.282	1.377	1.375	1.375	1.375	1.375	1.2
1.4	1.283	1.283	1.284	1.325	1.325	1.325	1.325	1.3
1.3	1.289	1.289	1.290	1.296	1.299	1.299	1.299	1.4
1.2	1.310	1.310	1.311	1.316	1.335	1.288	1.288	1.5
1.1	1.367	1.367	1.368	1.372	1.389	1.438	1.282	2.0
1.0	1.493	1.493	1.494	1.497	1.509	1.549	1.647	γ_2
	2.0	1.5	1.4	1.3	1.2	1.1	1.0	γ_1

$\begin{pmatrix} 1 & & \\ H & 1 & \\ H & L & 1 \end{pmatrix}$

$\begin{pmatrix} 1 & & \\ H & 1 & \\ M & M & 1 \end{pmatrix}$

γ_1	1.0	1.1	1.2	1.3	1.4	1.5	2.0	
γ_2	1.688	1.583	1.530	1.506	1.497	1.494	1.493	1.0
2.0	1.282	1.489	1.421	1.388	1.374	1.369	1.367	1.1
1.5	1.285	1.288	1.376	1.337	1.319	1.313	1.310	1.2
1.4	1.293	1.295	1.301	1.319	1.300	1.292	1.289	1.3
1.3	1.313	1.314	1.319	1.332	1.294	1.287	1.283	1.4
1.2	1.356	1.357	1.359	1.368	1.395	1.286	1.282	1.5
1.1	1.437	1.438	1.439	1.443	1.460	1.507	1.282	2.0
1.0	1.577	1.577	1.577	1.579	1.586	1.613	1.688	γ_2
	2.0	1.5	1.4	1.3	1.2	1.1	1.0	γ_1

$\begin{pmatrix} 1 & & \\ H & 1 & \\ M & M & 1 \end{pmatrix}$

(continued)

Table C.2 (continued)

$\rho = \begin{pmatrix} 1 & & \\ L & 1 & \\ M & M & 1 \end{pmatrix}$

γ_1	1.0	1.1	1.2	1.3	1.4	1.5	2.0	
γ_2	1.749	1.665	1.627	1.613	1.608	1.607	1.607	1.0
2.0	1.282	1.550	1.498	1.475	1.467	1.464	1.463	1.1
1.5	1.285	1.289	1.423	1.393	1.381	1.377	1.375	1.2
1.4	1.293	1.297	1.304	1.348	1.333	1.327	1.325	1.3
1.3	1.313	1.316	1.323	1.340	1.309	1.302	1.299	1.4
1.2	1.356	1.358	1.364	1.379	1.413	1.291	1.288	1.5
1.1	1.437	1.439	1.443	1.454	1.482	1.542	1.282	2.0
1.0	1.577	1.578	1.580	1.587	1.607	1.654	1.749	γ_2
	2.0	1.5	1.4	1.3	1.2	1.1	1.0	γ_1

$\begin{pmatrix} 1 & & \\ M & 1 & \\ M & L & 1 \end{pmatrix}$

$\begin{pmatrix} 1 & & \\ H & 1 & \\ L & L & 1 \end{pmatrix}$

γ_1	1.0	1.1	1.2	1.3	1.4	1.5	2.0	
γ_2	1.718	1.606	1.544	1.513	1.500	1.495	1.493	1.0
2.0	1.282	1.514	1.439	1.398	1.379	1.371	1.367	1.1
1.5	1.288	1.295	1.394	1.348	1.325	1.315	1.310	1.2
1.4	1.299	1.303	1.311	1.331	1.306	1.295	1.289	1.3
1.3	1.325	1.327	1.332	1.349	1.301	1.289	1.283	1.4
1.2	1.375	1.376	1.379	1.389	1.419	1.288	1.282	1.5
1.1	1.463	1.464	1.465	1.470	1.487	1.536	1.282	2.0
1.0	1.607	1.607	1.607	1.609	1.616	1.644	1.718	γ_2
	2.0	1.5	1.4	1.3	1.2	1.1	1.0	γ_1

$\begin{pmatrix} 1 & & \\ L & 1 & \\ L & H & 1 \end{pmatrix}$

$\begin{pmatrix} 1 & & \\ M & 1 & \\ L & L & 1 \end{pmatrix}$

γ_1	1.0	1.1	1.2	1.3	1.4	1.5	2.0	
γ_2	1.764	1.666	1.614	1.591	1.581	1.578	1.577	1.0
2.0	1.282	1.559	1.493	1.460	1.446	1.440	1.437	1.1
1.5	1.288	1.294	1.427	1.387	1.368	1.360	1.356	1.2
1.4	1.299	1.305	1.314	1.350	1.328	1.318	1.313	1.3
1.3	1.325	1.329	1.337	1.357	1.310	1.299	1.293	1.4
1.2	1.375	1.378	1.384	1.400	1.436	1.292	1.285	1.5
1.1	1.463	1.465	1.469	1.480	1.507	1.565	1.282	2.0
1.0	1.607	1.607	1.609	1.615	1.633	1.676	1.764	γ_2
	2.0	1.5	1.4	1.3	1.2	1.1	1.0	γ_1

$\begin{pmatrix} 1 & & \\ L & 1 & \\ L & M & 1 \end{pmatrix}$

$\begin{pmatrix} 1 & & \\ 0 & 1 & \\ M & M & 1 \end{pmatrix}$

γ_1	1.0	1.1	1.2	1.3	1.4	1.5	2.0	
γ_2	1.759	1.682	1.648	1.637	1.633	1.632	1.632	1.0
2.0	1.282	1.561	1.514	1.495	1.488	1.486	1.486	1.1
1.5	1.285	1.289	1.434	1.406	1.396	1.393	1.392	1.2
1.4	1.293	1.297	1.304	1.356	1.342	1.337	1.336	1.3
1.3	1.313	1.316	1.323	1.340	1.314	1.308	1.305	1.4
1.2	1.356	1.358	1.364	1.380	1.415	1.294	1.291	1.5
1.1	1.437	1.439	1.443	1.455	1.485	1.547	1.282	2.0
1.0	1.577	1.578	1.580	1.589	1.611	1.661	1.759	γ_2
	2.0	1.5	1.4	1.3	1.2	1.1	1.0	γ_1

$\begin{pmatrix} 1 & & \\ M & 1 & \\ M & 0 & 1 \end{pmatrix}$

$\begin{pmatrix} 1 & & \\ 0 & 1 & \\ L & L & 1 \end{pmatrix}$

γ_1	1.0	1.1	1.2	1.3	1.4	1.5	2.0	
γ_2	1.792	1.704	1.661	1.642	1.635	1.633	1.632	1.0
2.0	1.282	1.588	1.530	1.503	1.491	1.487	1.486	1.1
1.5	1.288	1.294	1.452	1.417	1.401	1.395	1.392	1.2
1.4	1.299	1.305	1.316	1.368	1.348	1.340	1.336	1.3
1.3	1.325	1.330	1.339	1.361	1.320	1.310	1.305	1.4
1.2	1.375	1.379	1.387	1.405	1.444	1.297	1.291	1.5
1.1	1.463	1.466	1.471	1.485	1.518	1.581	1.282	2.0
1.0	1.607	1.608	1.611	1.621	1.644	1.695	1.792	γ_2
	2.0	1.5	1.4	1.3	1.2	1.1	1.0	γ_1

$\begin{pmatrix} 1 & & \\ L & 1 & \\ L & 0 & 1 \end{pmatrix}$

Appendix D
Software Programs for Sample Size Calculation for Continuous Co-primary Endpoints

D.1 The R Macro

We provide the R code (ver 2.11.0) to calculate the solution C_K of (4.6), (4.11) and (4.15). We here apply the C_K to the sample size formula (4.5) (R is a free software package that the user can download from http://www.r-project.org/). In advance, the user needs to install the package mvtnorm and then submit the following code on the R console:

```
CKsolution <- function(alpha,power,rho,gamma,a,K){
   if(det(rho) <= 0){print("no positive definite");break}
   library(mvtnorm)
   z_a = qnorm(1-alpha); ndel = 0.001; rn = round(runif(1)*1000);
#  # Initial estimation of CK
   CK = qmvnorm(power, corr=rho, tail="lower.tail")$quantile
#  # Begin: Newton-Raphson algorithm to find CK
   for(j in 1:1000){
      set.seed(rn)
      C1k = CK*gamma + z_a*(a[K]*gamma - a[1:(K-1)])
      pow1 = pmvnorm(lower=rep(-Inf,K), upper=c(C1k,CK), corr=rho)[1]
      G = power - pow1
         if(abs(G) < 0.00001 & G <= 0){break}
      F1k = rep(0,K-1)
      for(l in 1:(K-1)){
       vndel = rep(0,K-1); vndel[l] = ndel
       F1k[l] = pmvnorm(lower=c(rep(-Inf,l-1),C1k[l],rep(-Inf,K-1)),
                     upper=c(C1k+vndel,CK), corr=rho)[1]/ndel }
         FK = pmvnorm(lower=c(rep(-Inf,K-1),CK),upper=c(C1k,CK+ndel),corr=rho)[1]/ndel
      dG = -t(F1k)%*%gamma - FK
      CK = CK - G/dG }
#  # End: Newton-Raphson algorithm to find CK
   return(c(CK))}}
```

The function named CKsolution has five arguments, alpha, power, rho, gamma, a and K, corresponding to α, $1 - \beta$, ρ, γ, $(a_1, \ldots, a_K)$ and K in this section, respectively. Note $a_1 = \cdots = a_K = 1$ is used for continuous endpoints. The part of the NR algorithm written in the above function code of CKsolution can be replaced by the "optimize" function equipped in the R.

The following example represents an application where $K = 2$, $\gamma = 8/7$, $\rho^{12} = 0.5$, $\alpha = 0.025$ and $\beta = 0.8$. The output, CKsolution[1]=0.9988124, is the solution $C_K(\beta, \rho, \gamma, \alpha)$ of (4.6). If $\delta = (0.4, 0.35)^T$ and $r = 1$, then n computed from (4.5) is

T. Sozu et al., *Sample Size Determination in Clinical Trials with Multiple Endpoints*, SpringerBriefs in Statistics, DOI 10.1007/978-3-319-22005-5

$$n \doteq 2(0.9988124 + z_{0.025})^2/0.35^2 \doteq 142.93 \to 143.$$

```
> K=2                                    # Specify by user
> a=c(1,1)                               # Specify by user
> gamma = c(8/7)                         # Specify by user
> rho<-matrix(c(  1 ,   0.5 ,            # Specify by user
+                 0.5 ,    1 ), ncol=K)
> CKsolution(0.025,0.8,rho,gamma,a,K)
[1]   0.9988124
```

The next example represents an application where $K = 3$, $\delta = (0.5, 0.45, 0.4)^{\mathrm{T}}$, $\rho^{12} = 0.8$, $\rho^{13} = 0.8$, $\rho^{23} = 0.5$, $\alpha = 0.025$ and $\beta = 0.8$. Then, using the output, CKsolution[1]= 1.018097, and the formula (4.5), the equal sample sizes per group $n = n_{\mathrm{T}} = n_{\mathrm{C}}$ (i.e., $r = 1.0$) is

$$n \doteq 2(1.018097 + z_{0.025})^2/0.4^2 \doteq 110.86 \to 111.$$

```
> K=3                                        # Specify by user
> delt1 = 0.5;  delt2 = 0.45;  delt3 = 0.4   # Specify by user
> a=c(1,1,1)                                 # Specify by user
> rho<-matrix(c(  1 , 0.8 , 0.8 ,            # Specify by user
+                 0.8 ,   1 , 0.5 ,
+                 0.8 , 0.5 ,   1), ncol=K)
> gamma = c(delt1/delt3, delt2/delt3)
> CKsolution(0.025,0.8,rho,gamma,a,K)
[1]   1.018097
```

D.2   The SAS Code

We provide the SAS code (ver 9.3) to calculate the solution C_K of (4.6). In advance, the user needs to download the macro MVN_DIST.sas (Genz 1992), http://www.biopharmnet.com/doc/doc14004d.sas and then submit the following code. This includes an application where $K = 3$, $\gamma = (1.25, 1.1)$, $\rho^{12} = 0.8$, $\rho^{13} = 0.5$ and $\rho^{23} = 0.3$ with $\alpha = 0.025$ and $\beta = 0.8$, where the inputs provided by the user are alpha, power, rho, gamma and vr corresponding to α, $1 - \beta$, ρ, γ and $(a_1, \ldots, a_K)$ in this section, respectively, and $a_1 = \cdots = a_K = 1$ is used for continuous endpoints.

```
proc iml;
%include"C:\MVN_DIST.sas";   * Specify a path where "MVN_DIST.sas" is located by user;
***** Begin Input by user;
    alpha = 0.025; power = 0.8;
    gamma = {1.25, 1.1};
    rho = { 1    0.8  0.5,
            0.8   1   0.3,
            0.5  0.3  1 };
    vr = {1, 1, 1};
***** End Input;
  K = nrow(rho);
  * calculation of CK;
  z_a = Quantile("Normal", 1-alpha); ndel = 0.001;
  CK = Quantile("Normal", power); * initial value of CK ;
  do until (abs(G) < 0.00001 & G <= 0);
  C1k = ck * gamma + z_a * (vr[K]*gamma - vr[1:K-1]);
  lower = J(1, K, 0);  upper = t(C1k) || CK;  infin = J(1, K, 0);
  maxpts = 4000*K*K*K;  abseps = 0.0001;  releps = 0;
  run mvn_dist(K,lower,upper,infin,rho,maxpts,abseps,releps,error,pow1,nevals,inform);
  G = power - pow1;
  F = J(1, K-1, 0);
  do l = 1 to K-1;
    vndel = J(1, K-1, 0); vndel[1,l] = ndel;
```

```
  infin = j(1, K ,0);    infin[1,1] = 2;
  lower = t(C1k) || CK;  upper = t(C1k) + vndel || CK;
 run mvn_dist(K,lower,upper,infin,rho,maxpts,abseps,releps,error,value,nevals,inform);
 F[1] = value / ndel;
 end;
 lower = t(C1k) || CK;  upper = t(C1k) || CK + ndel;
 infin = J(1, K ,0);
 infin[1,K] = 2;
 run mvn_dist(K,lower,upper,infin,rho,maxpts,abseps,releps,error,value,nevals,inform);
 FK = value / ndel;
 dG = -F*gamma - FK;
 CK = CK - G/dG;
 end;
 print CK;
quit;
```

Reference

Genz A Numerical computation of multivariate normal probabilities. J Comput Graph Stat 1:141–150 (1992)

Printed in the United States
By Bookmasters